Sugar

and the

Evil Empire

How Multi-National Food Companies Have
Turned The Western Population Into
Sugar Addicts

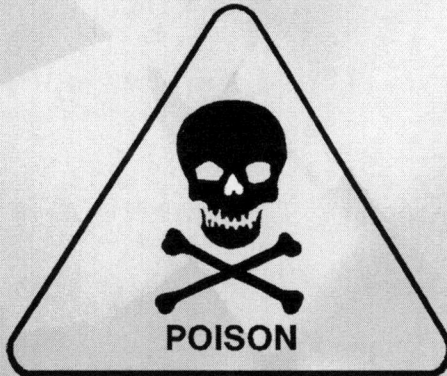

POISON

A Terra Novian Report

Geoff & Vicky Wells

Cover Design: Geoff Wells

PAPERBACK EDITION 2014

Manufactured in the United States of America

CreateSpace Independent Publishing Platform

ISBN-13: 978-1499332827
ISBN-10: 1499332823

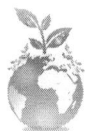

TERRA NOVIAN PRESS

MIAMI
TORONTO

http://www.terranovian.com

Dedication

To all the people throughout history who lost their freedom, their health or their lives so that others could profit from their misfortune.

We would like to believe those times are over but they are not. The rich and powerful 1% are becoming more unscrupulous every day.

Table of Contents

SECTION 2 MEDICAL

Section 3 Sugar Addiction

Section 4
Corporate Complicity

Section 5 Living With Sugar

An Introduction to a Sugar Free Diet?

Section 6 Cooking Without Sugar

Section 7 Recap

SECTION 8 BEFORE YOU GO

SECTION 8 INDEX

A Personal Message

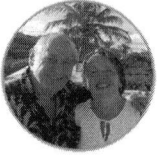

We are not scientist, we're just ordinary people that have been lied to our whole lives. Some of the lies were mistakes but many were and are deliberate.

We may not be scientists but we can read and we have the time to sort out the truth from the lies. You can easily check what we have written by visiting the links we provide or, better still, do your own research.

If you find any errors they are ours. The science is solid and for your sake, your children's sake and the sake of future generations you need to believe it and do something about it.

This is not a book full of exhaustive scientific proof, it is a book of conclusions that you can make use of immediately. We share our resources and encourage you to check them out. Just don't wait until you have the time to check them before you make some changes to your diet.

We have done our best to present what we have learned in an approachable and understandable way. We have also incorporated what we've learned into our own lives and we are starting to reap the benefits of our new lifestyle.

We've lost weight and gained energy, our blood analysis is green across the board and our general health is excellent.

We grow most of our own food and delight in the wonderful flavours that we have not tasted since we were kids.

We hope you will find the time to visit our web site and look at some of the other important topics we have discovered.

http://terranovian.com

There is nothing you need to buy or sign up for, just solid information. If you discover some disconcerting topic you didn't even know you should be concerned about, then we have done our job.

Geoff & Vicky Wells
The first Terra Novians

Who Are The Evil Empire?

We will make repeated references throughout this book to "The Evil Empire" so we should first make clear who we are referring to.

The Evil Empire are the 1% of the population that control the wealth and power of the planet. The politicians, industrialists and bankers that have built their fortunes on the backs of others. Old money that is passed down from generation to generation and used to influence public opinion, pervert justice and ensure the continued existence of the privileged few.

These are people that worship profit above all else. They have no regard for human rights, the environment or future generations. They live to generate profit, here and now, no matter what the consequences.

It is our opinion that the relentless quest for more profit will inevitably deplete all planetary resources and lead to the extinction of the human race.

This has nothing to do with conspiracies, it is a simple application of mathematics. There can be no argument that if we continue to use finite resources we must, at some point, run out, The only argument is when this will happen and the severity of the repercussions when it does.

This book is more focused on the consequences to our health from believing the lies of the packaged food industry than it is on the squandering of precious resources. But make no mistake, the cost of the damage being done to our farmlands, the indiscriminate tampering with the genetic code of our seeds and the total disregard for the health of our bees must, one day, be paid.

The path followed by western society believes that possessions equal happiness and that the people with the most possessions are therefore the happiest - this is "The American Dream". This path is now a super highway leading us to our destruction. We must change our way while there is still time

Follow the Terra Novian Way

http://terranovian.com

SECTION 1
IT BEGINS WITH GRASS

Sugar has a 3,000 year history of creating wealth and misery. In our time it has added obesity to its list of credits.

We begin the story 10,000 years ago, in Asia.

The History of Sugar

Sugar has been around for a long time - over 10,000 years. It is a tropical grass that was first domesticated in New Guinea and the natives there, like growers today, would pick and chew the cane to get at the sweet juice.

Although modern man evolved around 200,000 years ago, agriculture has only existed for about 10,000 years. This makes sugar one of the first crops to be grown.

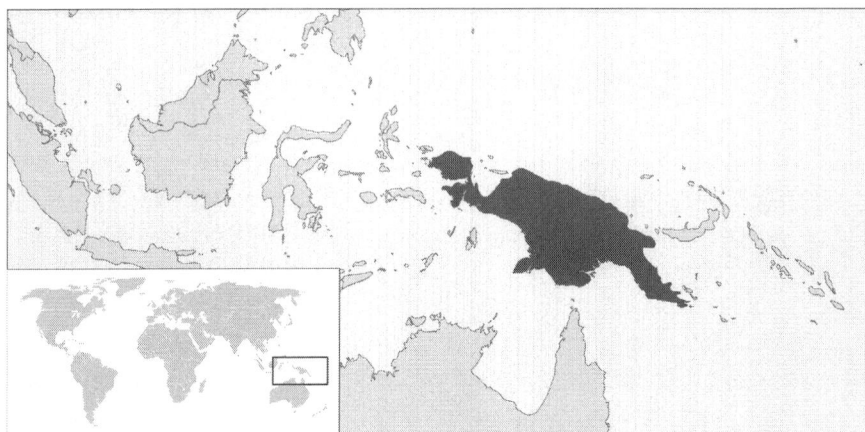

New Guinea is just South and East of Thailand but it wasn't until about 1000 B.C. that sugar finally reached the main continent of Asia.

By 500 A.D. the Indians had learned how to process the cane into a powder which was used as a medicine to cure headaches, stomach aches and impotence.

The art of sugar refining was a closely guarded secret but by 600 A.D. it had spread to Persia (modern day Iran) where the rulers provided all kinds of sweets for their guests. When the Arab armies conquered the area they acquired the refining secret and spread the knowledge across the Muslim world.

For the Caliphs, sugar, and even more so, marzipan, which is sugar mixed with ground almonds, was used as a display of their wealth. They would commission elaborate sculptures made of marzipan which, once admired, were eaten by the poor.

The Arabs perfected the sugar refining process but the work was hard and hot, only suitable for slaves. The slaves were primarily eastern European soldiers captured in the Muslim / Christian battles.

British and French crusaders, fighting in the Holy Land, were the first Westerners to come under the spell of sugar. Unfortunately, French and British climates are not suitable for growing large quantities of sugar cane so only a small market could be built from the minimal quantities acquired from Muslim traders.

Sugar was so rare in the western world that it was considered a spice. Only the wealthy nobility could afford what little there was. The spread of the Ottoman empire in the 1400s dried up what little trade there was with the Muslims.

This did not sit well with the Western nobility but, since sugar cane needs a wet, tropical climate to flourish, the only alternatives were to defeat the Muslims or find somewhere else to grow their sugar.

THE AGE OF EXPLORATION

The 1400s was a period in history that saw European explorers searching the globe for new lands. This expansion was driven in no small measure by the search for land to grow sugar cane.

The Portuguese planted cane in Madeira and the other newly discovered Atlantic islands of Cape Verde and the Canaries soon followed.

Sugar production was immensely profitable but required a large labor force. The Portuguese were already involved in slaves, gold, ivory and pepper trade with Africa, so bringing the slaves to the nearby islands to cultivate sugar cane was an obvious step.

On his second voyage to the Americas in 1493, Christopher Columbus planted sugar cane in Hispaniola, today's Haiti and the Dominican Republic. In his youth he had lived on Madeira and trained in the sugar trade.

THE EVIL EMPIRE BEGINS

Priests and nobility have been the ruling classes since the dawn of history. There has never been any torture too severe or punishment not enacted by this small group upon their fellow man. Wealth, power and religion is the motivation and justification for every unspeakable act throughout history.

With the rise of the sugar trade came the opportunity for those on the fringes of the ruling class, if they were ruthless enough, to acquire their share of the new wealth and power.

Not only the aristocracy, but traders and land owners of all sorts, were about to get very rich - never mind the price.

SLAVERY

Sugar cane quickly spread throughout the Caribbean and into South America. The native populations were either enslaved or killed in combat or by diseases for which they had no immunity.

Over the next several centuries the plantations expanded, the price of sugar dropped and demand increased. By the middle of the 17th century even the European poor had added sugar to their diet. The demand for sugar was enormous and so was the demand for new slaves.

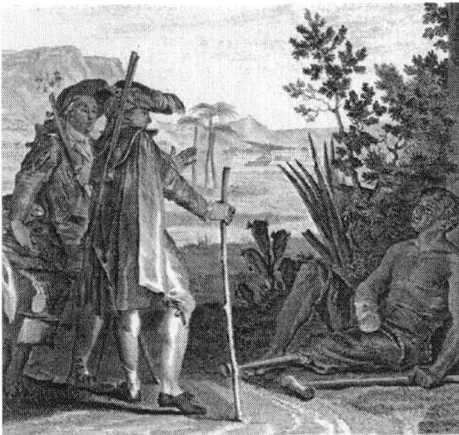

This engraving is from Voltaire's Candide: it depicts the scene where Candide and Cacambo meet a maimed slave of a sugar mill near Surinam. Its caption reads in English, "It is at this price that you eat sugar in Europe"; this line was said by the slave in the text. The "negro" has had his hand cut off for getting a finger stuck in a millstone and his leg removed for trying to run away.

Each new sugar crop meant another round of misery for the Africans. The sugar was sold in the markets of London, Paris and Amsterdam where the ships would load up with products to be traded in Africa for more slaves.

Tribal conflicts guaranteed there would always be prisoners that could be traded to the slavers. It must be remembered that slavery was an African institution long before the Europeans arrived. People, rather than land, was the basis for wealth among the Africans.

By the beginning of the 1800s more than 11 million Africans had made the journey to the Americas, half of them ending up in the sugar plantations.

Millions of lives were lost so that Europeans could eat a few sweets and have sugar for their tea. Eventually the public learned of the abuses and began protesting against the inhuman treatment. Many boycotted sugar made by slave labor and, by voting with their cash, forced the Evil Empire to change their practises.

Much the same is happening today over the GMO debate and many of the major food companies are being forced to remove GM food from products destined to countries which have anti-GMO legislation.

The British Slave Trade Act of 1807 outlawed the practice of slave trading but not slavery itself. In an effort to enforce the act, the Royal Navy began patrolling the West Coast of Africa but with terrible consequences. A captain in danger of being caught would sometimes simply throw the slaves overboard rather than pay the fine.

A widely held belief is that British slavery ended when Britain enacted the Slavery Abolition Act of 1833, but this is only partially true. Of course it only applied to British colonies and not all of them were included. Any territories in the possession of the East India Company, and the island of Ceylon, and the island of Saint Helena were exempt. Slavery in India was not abolished until 1843.

Also, the law only applied to slaves under the age of six. Those over the age of six were simply redesignated as "apprentices" and forced to continue working in exchange for free board and lodging.

Full emancipation was not achieved until August 1st, 1838.

It took quite a while for slavery to actually end. Even after Britain made the practice illegal, it was another 27 years before the US did.

In the United States slavery was abolished by the thirteenth amendment to the constitution. The amendment was passed by the Senate in April 1864, the House of Representatives in January 1865 but did not take effect until it was ratified by three quarters of the States in December 1865.

However, even though slavery became illegal in the United States, in a lot of cases it was replaced by indentured servitude. So, initially, not much actually changed.

THE EVIL EMPIRE NEVER LOSES

Laws, of course, are made by those with the wealth and power and many of the wealthy and powerful of the time were slave owners. The British Act compensated slave-owners for their lose of "property" to the tune of Twenty Million Pounds Stirling. That's equivalent to over 33 billion in US dollars today.

Not surprisingly, the slaves themselves got absolutely nothing.

You can see exactly who benefited and by how much by looking through the database at:

http://www.ucl.ac.uk/lbs/

For many former slave owners the investment of these windfall funds formed the basis of family fortunes that continue today.

SUGAR BEETS

The importance of sugar cane has gradually declined as sugar beet production has taken its place. Sugar beets now account for more than 20% of the world's production.

The sugar beet, which is related to beetroot and Swiss chard, are all descendents of the wild sea beet. Sugar beets contain a high concentration of sucrose but, unlike sugar cane, they can be grown in regions of Europe and North America that meet the particular growing conditions that are required.

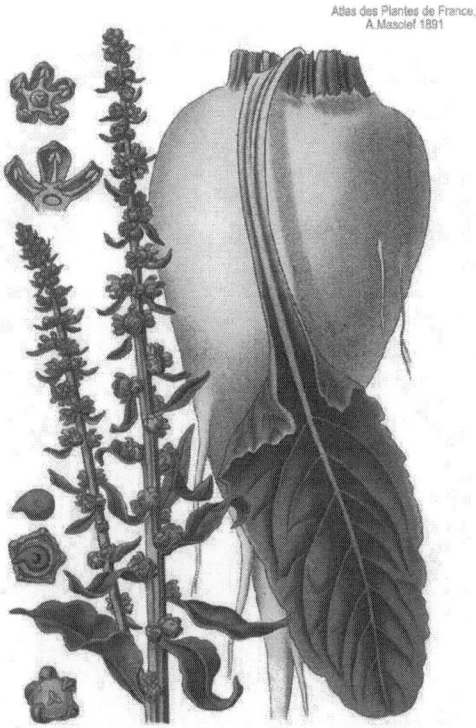

Atlas des Plantes de France.
A.Masclef 1891

Pl.276. *Bette vulgaire.(Betterave).* Beta vulgaris L.

Although the properties of the sugar beet were known by the late 1700s, commercial production didn't begin until Napoleon Bonaparte compelled farmers to plant large acreages of them and prohibited the import of Caribbean sugar cane in 1813.

GENETIC MODIFICATION

The growing of Monsanto's genetically modified sugar beets is banned worldwide except for the USA and Canada. Like most of Monsanto's mutations, they are designed to be resistant to the herbicide Glyphosate, which is the chemical name for Monsanto's Roundup. The sales pitch for Roundup-ready GM beets is that farmers will get higher yields and use fewer chemicals. Roundup can be sprayed on the GM sugar beets to kill weeds without killing the beets. It's a good theory but in practice the reality is that the weeds also develop an immunity to the Glyphosate and the farmer has to spray more and more chemicals on our food in order to kill the weeds.

Consumers in the USA and Canada therefore face, not only all the problems associated with sugar consumption, but also unknown dangers from ingesting genetically altered foods and the toxic effects of chemical residues that cause the [1]destruction of red blood cells, lung dysfunction, low blood pressure, kidney damage, erosion of gastrointestinal tract, dizziness, fever, and nausea.

THE EVIL EMPIRE WINS AGAIN

Monsanto is the poster child for the Evil Empire. If not stopped they may become responsible for the genocide of the human race, but the Monsanto story is beyond the scope of this book. If you wish to learn more visit:

  http://terranovian.com/food/gmo.html

In regards to Monsanto and GM sugar beets, various lawsuits have been brought against Monsanto and, for a brief time, they were declared unlawful and farmers were not allowed to grow them. Unfortunately, money and influence won out and as of July 2012 the USDA deregulated Monsanto's Roundup-ready sugar beets.

Monsanto spends millions of dollars in efforts to defeat campaigns that are trying to have GM ingredients identified on product labels. Until such time as the US and Canada catches up with Europe's labeling laws, we urge you to look for the Non GMO Project labels on foods you suspect may contain GMO ingredients.

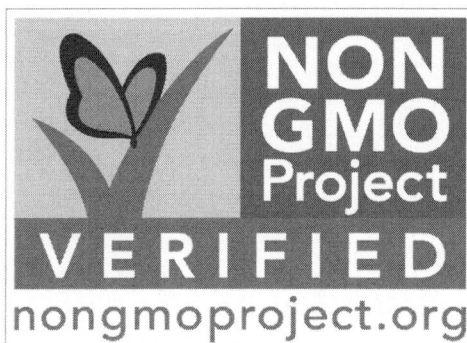

NON GMO Project VERIFIED
nongmoproject.org

---

1   http://www.sierraclub.ca/national/programs/health-environment/ pesticides/Glyphosate-fact-sheet.shtml

Sugar Cane Today

Much of today's sugar cane is still grown using cheap labor in countries that allow, or at least turn a blind eye to, the exploitation of workers. Children in the Philippines, Kenya, and Bolivia, some as young as 6, toil in the hot sun pulling weeds in seven and eight hour shifts.

Workers in El Salvador, Nicaragua, India and Sri Lanka spray dangerous chemicals without the benefit of protective clothing and suffer the consequences of an early death due to liver failure.

Chronic Kidney Disease (or CKD) is considered an epidemic throughout South and Central America. It kills more young men than HIV/AIDS, diabetes and leukemia combined.

To add insult to injury, in Nicaragua, the Nicaragua Sugar Estates Limited (NSEL) fires any workers that test positive for CKD. For these workers it means the end of family income. The only alternative is for the wives and children to work in the fields.

ETHANOL PRODUCTION

Plans by the major industrialized nations to expand the use of ethanol fuels to combat climate change will further exacerbate the workers problems as demand for sugar cane will rise.

High Fructose Corn Syrup

[2]Corn syrup is often confused with High Fructose Corn Syrup. Corn syrup is made from corn starch and is not particularly sweet.

[3]High Fructose Corn Syrup (HFCS) was originally developed in Japan between 1965 and 1970. It is made by converting much of the glucose in corn syrup to the much sweeter fructose.

Before the dawn of HFCS, our exposure to fructose was limited to the consumption of fruits such as grapes, apples, blueberries, etc. Most fruits are only 5-10% fructose by weight and come with many other benefits such as fiber and beneficial nutrients.

Molasses and common dried fruits have a content of less than 10% fructose.

The staples of many diets - milk, meat, fresh vegetables, fresh fruits - prior to the introduction of HFCS and highly processed foods, contained little to no fructose.

Government subsidies have made corn profitable to grow and very cheap to use as a food additive.

Since the 1970s there has been more than a 25% increase in "added sugars" in our processed and packaged foods. Much of that added sugar is fructose.

[4]A recent study has found that countries that consume a diet high in HFCS have 20% more cases of type 2 diabetes than countries that do not.

To make a bad situation even worse, HFCS is made from GMO corn. This same corn is fed to cattle which makes them sick so they must be injected with antibiotics which, of course, ends up in our steaks, ribs and Sunday roast. Is it any wonder everyone is getting sick?

---

2   http://en.wikipedia.org/wiki/Corn_syrup
3   http://en.wikipedia.org/wiki/High_fructose_corn_syrup
4   http://pressroom.usc.edu/researchers-at-university-of-southern-california-and-university-of-oxford-find-link-between-high-fructose-corn-syrup-and-increased-global-prevalence-of-diabetes/

Secretary of Agriculture Earl Butz

[5]Earl Butz was the US Secretary of Agriculture under Presidents Richard Nixon and Gerald Ford. It was his policies that brought about the rise of large agribusiness corporations, the end of small family farms and, ultimately, the current obesity crisis.

After the Great Depression, President Franklin D. Roosevelt introduced a series of programs dubbed "[6]The New Deal". The programs were designed to offer relief to the poor and unemployed, recovery of the economy and reform of the laws that had allowed Wall Street to rape the middle class.

As part of the new deal the [7]Agricultural Adjustment Act of 1933 was introduced under then Secretary of Agriculture, [8]Vice President Henry A. Wallace.

The Agricultural Adjustment Act was a way to raise the price farmers received for their produce. Basically, farmers were paid by the government to remove acreage from production which lowered the supply of certain items, such as corn, and raised the prices.

The program was seen as largely successful for small farmers but many itinerant laborers, primarily black, lost their livelihood due to diminished demand.

During his tenure as Secretary of Agriculture from 1971 to 1976, Earl Butz abolished the program that paid farmers not to plant corn and instead encouraged farmers to grow as much as possible.

Farmers are now insured against loss from environmental disasters and also from low prices due to overproduction. In this win-win situation huge agribusiness corporations have taken over from the small farmer and are producing more and more crops that we can't use.

In an effort to get rid of all the corn we produce it gets turned into High Fructose Corn Syrup, gets fed to cattle instead of grass and gets turned into

5   http://en.wikipedia.org/wiki/Earl_Butz
6   http://en.wikipedia.org/wiki/New_Deal
7   http://en.wikipedia.org/wiki/Agricultural_Adjustment_Act
8   http://en.wikipedia.org/wiki/Henry_A._Wallace

ethanol fuel which many experts believe takes more energy to produce than it contains.

Now that China and the European Union have refused to import GMO corn there will be an even bigger surplus in the years to come.

What Your Sugar Habit Supports

In reality, little has changed since the days of slavery. Spend a little time investigating the links below to discover the abuses sugar purchases support.

A CYCLE OF DEATH: INSIDE NICARAGUA'S SUGAR CANE FIELDS

http://upsidedownworld.org/main/nicaragua-archives-62/3402-a-cycle-of-death-inside-nicaraguas-sugar-cane-fields

MYSTERY KIDNEY DISEASE DECIMATES CENTRAL AMERICA SUGARCANE WORKERS

http://investigations.nbcnews.com/_news/2012/10/16/13866856-mystery-kidney-disease-decimates-central-america-sugarcane-workers?lite

EXPLOITATION OF WORKERS IN THE DOMINICAN REPUBLIC'S SUGAR FIELDS CONTINUES

http://www.aflcio.org/Blog/Global-Action/Exploitation-of-Workers-in-the-Dominican-Republic-s-Sugar-Fields-Continues

WHAT IS KILLING SUGAR-CANE WORKERS ACROSS CENTRAL AMERICA?

http://www.theguardian.com/world/2012/oct/14/kidney-disease-killing-sugar-cane-workers-central-america

LIFE NOT SWEET FOR PHILIPPINES' SUGAR CANE CHILD WORKERS

http://edition.cnn.com/2012/05/01/world/asia/

philippines-child-labor/

THOUSANDS OF SUGAR CANE WORKERS DIE AS WEALTHY NATIONS STALL ON SOLUTIONS

http://www.publicintegrity.org/2011/12/12/7578/
thousands-sugar-cane-workers-die-wealthy-nations-
stall-solutions

SUGARCANE WORKERS PLAN TO STOP CHILD-LABOUR

http://www.africasciencenews.org/en/index.
php?option=com_content&view=article&id
=665:sugarcane-workers-plan-to-stop-child-
labour&catid=49:food&Itemid=113

YALE SENIOR TAKES ON THE PLIGHT OF NICARAGUAN SUGAR WORKERS

http://news.yale.edu/2013/05/01/spotlight-yale-senior-
takes-plight-nicaraguan-sugar-workers

CHILD LABOR IN SUGARCANE

http://endchildlabor.org/?cat=121

SECTION 2 MEDICAL

We've always had the sense that sugar wasn't good for us but it's only recently that science has discovered exactly why sugar is bad and just how bad it is.

In this section we look at how our bodies are affected by sugar and also many of the other factors in our diet that are contributing to the obesity epidemic.

By no means does this section contain all there is to know on the subject but we have tried to include all we need to know. If you discover areas you wish to investigate further, or issues you did not know existed, then we have done our job.

We are only skimming the surface of nutritional science and new discoveries are being made every day. Please use the references we have provided to learn more.

When Is A Calorie Not A Calorie?

There are two measurements called a calorie, large calorie and small calorie. Each one is a measurement of heat in degrees Celsius but the measurement scale is different.

[1]The small calorie or gram calorie (symbol: cal) is the approximate amount of energy needed to raise the temperature of one gram of water by one degree Celsius.

The large calorie, kilogram calorie, dietary calorie, nutritionist's calorie or food calorie (symbol: Cal, equiv: kcal) is the amount of energy needed to raise the temperature of one kilogram of water by one degree Celsius. The large calorie is thus equal to 1000 small calories or one kilocalorie (symbol: kcal).

If you are reading this in Europe you are probably more familiar with [2]food energy being expressed in joules (J) or kilojoules (kJ) but what we are about to say applies equally to you.

An often quoted maxim is that "A calorie is a calorie", but this is just not true. The idea is that it doesn't matter where our calories come from, donuts or apples, ice cream or nuts, soft drinks or milk - the result is the same. This is what we have been taught for years, but it's a lie.

From the scientific heat energy perspective the maxim is true but, from our body's perspective, there is a tremendous difference between drinking 120 calories of a soft drink and eating 120 calories of bread.

The difference is that half the calories in a soft drink come from the sugar fructose and the calories in the bread come from the sugar glucose. It's all about how our bodies process the two sugars and how each affects our weight.

This is what all the attention is about in regards to Dr. Lustig's YouTube video.

---

1   http://en.wikipedia.org/wiki/Calorie
2   http://en.wikipedia.org/wiki/Food_energy

Dr. Robert Lustig

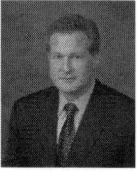

[3]Sugar: The Bitter Truth - a YouTube video by Dr. Robert Lustig - has been viewed more than 4 million times. The current anti-sugar movement, this, and many other books owe their existence to this viral video.

The 90-minute video manages to explain the very complicated processes of human metabolism in a humorous and entertaining way. Dr. Lustig's presentation is light and easily understandable. If you want to truly understand the role sugar plays in obesity, heart disease, diabetes and cancer, you need to find the time to watch it.

We attempt to summarize, briefly, the main points presented in the video so that you are able to understand the balance of this book, even if you have not had the opportunity to view it.

All the scientific data is available by following the links we have provided, so we will not be covering the detailed scientific information in Dr. Lustig's video.

We also recommended watching a second video from Dr. Lustig entitled [4]Fat Chance: Fructose 2.0, which is also available on YouTube or you can watch them both from the Terra Novian web site.

http://www.terranovian.com/food/sugar.html

Dr. Lustig has also released a book based on the material in his two lectures called "Fat Chance". Although the videos, as well as the book, can be understood and enjoyed by the general public, they also contain a great deal of medical information that is directed more to medical professionals.

Much of what is included in this book comes from the work of Dr. Lustig, however, we focus more on the conclusions than on the science behind those conclusions.

Keep in mind, as you read this book, the research is available for those who wish to delve deeper into the subject.

---

3   http://www.terranovian.com/food/sugar.html
4   http://www.terranovian.com/food/sugar.html

[5]CARBOHYDRATES

Carbohydrates are types of sugars or saccharides, basically, large biological molecules of carbon, hydrogen and oxygen.

Sugar is divided into four groups; [6]monosaccharides, [7]disaccharides, [8]oligosaccharides and [9]polysaccharides. Monosaccharides are the base sugars. Disaccharides are various combinations of two base sugars. Oligosaccharides contain between three and nine monosaccharides. Polysaccharides are long chains of hundreds or thousands of monosaccharides.

The monosaccharides are glucose, fructose and galactose. These are combined in various ways to form the disaccharides sucrose, lactose and maltose.

Carbohydrates are essential to life and perform many roles in living organisms from energy storage to the cellulose structure of plants and the exoskeleton (chitin) of arthropods.

Carbohydrates are part of the genetic molecule RNA and a component of DNA. They are also key players in the immune system, fertilization, preventing pathogenesis, blood clotting, and development.

In this book we look at carbohydrates in the context of food science which refers to carbohydrates as foods containing complex carbohydrate starch such as cereals, bread and pasta. And, of course, the main focus of the book is the simple carbohydrate, sugar.

BLOOD SUGAR

We each have around five and a half liters of blood in our bodies. That gallon and a bit of blood contains about one teaspoon of sugar - that's it. If the level of sugar in our blood rises to, say, one tablespoon, we go into a hyperglycemic coma and die.

---

5   http://en.wikipedia.org/wiki/Carbohydrate

6   http://en.wikipedia.org/wiki/Monosaccharide

7.   http://en.wikipedia.org/wiki/Disaccharide

8   http://en.wikipedia.org/wiki/Oligosaccharide

9   http://en.wikipedia.org/wiki/Polysaccharide

[10]Even a quarter teaspoonful will take us from normal to pre-diabetic. ([11]An average adult body with a weight of 150 to 180 pounds will contain approximately 4.7 to 5.5 liters (1.2 to 1.5 gallons) of blood.)

Starch (amylum)

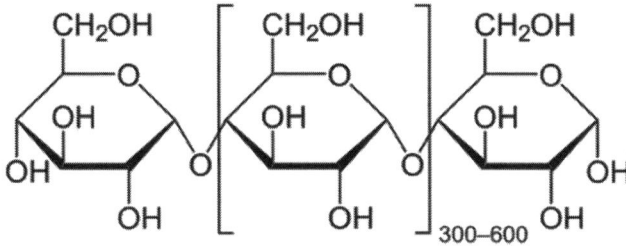

[12]Starch or amylum is a polysaccharide consisting of a large number of glucose units joined by glycosidic bonds. It is produced by most green plants as an energy store and is the most common carbohydrate in human diets.

The starch in potatoes, peas, corn and beans, etc and in any grains or grain products like bread, pasta or cereal, is digested by our bodies into glucose and fiber.

Our bodies can't break down the fiber but it plays a very important part in our digestion which we'll get to a little later.

DISACCHARIDES

The food industry has done a wonderful job of hiding added sugar by giving their ingredients a variety of creative names by which they fulfil labeling requirements.

Later in this book we provide a detailed list of the types and names of sugar frequently used on food labels. But in this section, we are only concerned with chemical sugars and how our bodies deal with them.

---

10   http://www.proteinpower.com/drmike/sugar-and-sweeteners/a-spoonful-of-sugar/

11   http://wonderopolis.org/wonder/how-much-blood-is-in-your-body/

12   http://en.wikipedia.org/wiki/Starch

[13]Sucrose (glucose-fructose)

Sucrose is the scientific name for the substance most of us refer to as table sugar. It's the white granules we put in our tea or coffee, sprinkle on our cereal and use to sweeten cakes, cookies, pies and some soft drinks.

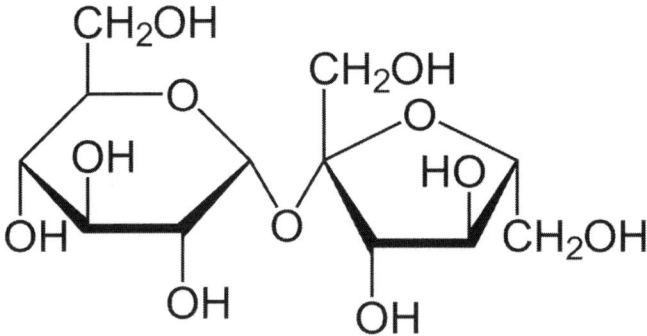

This stuff is in about 90% of the packaged and processed foods we pile into our shopping carts each week.

[14]The sucrose molecule is a disaccharide composed of the monosaccharides glucose and fructose.

In 2013, the worldwide production of sucrose was approximately 175 million metric tons.

[15]Lactose (Milk Sugar - glucose-galactose)

Lactose is the sugar found in breast milk, human or animal. Mammalian babies produce an enzyme called [16]lactase which is required to digest lactose. After weaning the majority of the human population stops producing lactase and ingesting lactose produces a condition called [17]lactose intolerance.

13   http://en.wikipedia.org/wiki/Sucrose
14   https://highered.mcgraw-hill.com/sites/0072507470/student_view0/chapter25/animation__enzyme_action_and_the_hydrolysis_of_sucrose.html
15   http://en.wikipedia.org/wiki/Lactose
16   http://en.wikipedia.org/wiki/Lactase
17   http://en.wikipedia.org/wiki/Lactose_intolerance

The ability to metabolize lactose as an adult evolved independently in many regions but is only present in [18]25-35% of the worldwide population - predominantly those of us with ancestry from [19]Europe, India, Arabia and parts of East Africa.

For those of us that can digest milk sugar, our liver turns it into glucose so it can be used directly as energy.

[20]Maltose (glucose-glucose),

Maltose is a disaccharide of glucose and glucose so our bodies can easily use it as energy.

It is found in beer, also in cereal, pasta, potatoes and the food industry uses it as a sweetener in many processed products.

MONOSACCHARIDES

[21]Glucose

Glucose alone is not very sweet. Try some corn syrup, such as Karo in the USA or Bee Hive in Canada, and you will taste pure glucose.

NOTE: This is very different to High Fructose Corn Syrup which we will get to later.

Glucose is the energy of life. It is used throughout the entire body to power various systems. Every living organism, from bacteria to humans, uses glucose for energy. As a matter of fact, if we don't get glucose from our food, our body makes it.

Glucose accounts for half of the sugar in sucrose. That means that 50% of the 15 calories in a teaspoon of table sugar comes from glucose, which is easily metabolized by all of the organs of the body. So, those 7.5 calories

---

18   http://genetics.thetech.org/original_news/news45

19   http://news.discovery.com/human/health/milk-drinking-still-a-mystery-140121.htm

20   http://en.wikipedia.org/wiki/Maltose

21   http://en.wikipedia.org/wiki/Glucose

are not only good for us but are actually needed by our body. The other 7.5 calories - not so much.

The majority of the glucose we eat is metabolized directly by all the cells in our body and the rest (about 20%) is metabolized by our liver. Even though it is good for us, any glucose we eat, over and above what we need to power our systems, gets stored as fat.

Glucose is found naturally in plants and other carbohydrates such as cereals, bread and pasta.

Glucose Metabolism
What does our body do with glucose?

As we said earlier, glucose is essential to life but we still don't want too much. Glucose is energy - period. That's why high starch foods are called "empty calories". We either burn it or store it for later.

In his video ,"Sugar: The Bitter Truth", Dr Lustig demonstrates what happens to 120 calories of the various monosaccharides. First we look at the 120 calories of glucose found in one-half cup of cooked white rice.

Twenty percent, or 24 calories is metabolized by our liver, the other 96 calories are burned by the mitochondria in our cells in what is called the [22]Krebs cycle which turns the glucose into carbon dioxide, water and energy.

If you really want to understand the process there is an excellent animation here:

https://highered.mcgraw-hill.com/sites/0072507470/student_view0/chapter25/animation__how_the_krebs_cycle_works__quiz_1_.html

A small amount of the glucose energy will be used by the liver itself as a power source but the majority of the 24 calories of glucose that enters the liver gets turned into glycogen (liver starch) which the liver stores as a quick source of energy. After a meal, the liver supplies our bodies with glucose from its store of glycogen.

---

22   http://en.wikipedia.org/wiki/Citric_acid_cycle

When our pancreas detects glucose in the bloodstream it releases insulin which directs our fat cells to open up and accept the glucose for long term storage.

So any of those 96 calories that don't get used right away get converted to triglycerides (fat) and float in our bloodstream until they get deposited as visceral fat around our waist.

Too much glucose will make us fat and if our visceral fat deposits grow our waistline to more than about 40" for men and 35" for women, then it's time to seriously consider a diet. But, otherwise, too much glucose is not harmful, not so much with fructose.

[23]*Fructose*

Fructose is sweet and the convenience food division of the Evil Empire adds it to all kinds of "food" to mask the taste of some of the other junk they mix in.

Fructose makes up the other 50% of sucrose (table sugar). This is the bad stuff that we have to eliminate from our diet or, at the very least, mitigate its effects with fiber.

It cannot be used by our body directly and must be metabolized (broken down) by our liver. It does not get used immediately and instead gets stored as visceral fat.

Fructose is also found naturally in fruits, berries and root vegetables but these natural foods also contain large quantities of dietary fiber.

Fructose Metabolism
What does our body do with fructose?

Instead of 120 calories of glucose from rice, we'll look at 120 calories of sucrose (50% glucose and 50% fructose) from an eight ounce glass of orange juice. Notice that the juice is just as bad as a soft drink.

The 120 calories is split 50/50 between glucose and fructose and the 60 glucose calories do the same 12 calories to the liver and 48 to the mitochondria split. Now comes the problem, the mitochondria cannot

23   http://en.wikipedia.org/wiki/Fructose

metabolize fructose so it all has to go to the liver for processing. 12 calories from the glucose and 60 calories from the fructose, that's 72 calories hitting the liver instead of the 24 calories it would get from glucose alone. That's three times as much from an equal calorie intake.

"So what," we may say, "it's still the same number of calories."

We started this section by asking "When is a calorie not a calorie?". This is the answer.

This gets a little technical so stay with us and we will try to sort out just enough to understand what's happening.

To start with, the extra load on the liver means it needs more energy to metabolize the fructose which leads to the depletion of [24]adenosine triphosphate (or [25]ATP, the vital chemical that conveys energy within cells). This depletion generates the waste product uric acid which causes gout and increases blood pressure.

[26]Unlike glucose, fructose does not get converted into glycogen, instead it is changed to acetyl-CoA which is an energy transport mechanism used by the mitochondria. What the mitochondria can't use gets stored as fat.

Fructose activates a liver enzyme that leads to liver insulin resistance which means there is less control over the amount of glucose the liver adds to the bloodstream.

This liver insulin resistance causes the pancreas to release more insulin which forces more energy to be stored as fat. This is the visceral fat that gets stored around our organs and adds inches to our belt size.

FRUCTOSE IS A CHRONIC POISON

Dr. Lustig offers a mountain of evidence, in both his videos and his books, along with very persuasive arguments to demonstrate that fructose is a poison. It's not an acute poison such as cyanide, which will kill us

24   http://en.wikipedia.org/wiki/Adenosine_triphosphate
25   https://highered.mcgraw-hill.com/sites/0072507470/student_view0/chapter25/animation__electron_transport_system_and_atp_syn-thesis__quiz_1_.html
26   http://en.wikipedia.org/wiki/Fructolysis

immediately. It's a chronic poison that takes years to do the job. But acute or chronic, either way, we end up just as dead.

Dr. Lustig also points out that, just as the tobacco branch of the Evil Empire was aware of the effects of cigarettes, the processed food branch is equally aware of the effects of sugar.

[27]Galactose (Dairy)

The monosaccharides glucose and galactose form lactose which is the sugar found in milk, human or animal. As long as our body is able to supply the enzyme [28]lactase, the galactose is rapidly processed into glucose and our body has no problem with glucose.

The problem, as usual, comes from, the Evil Empire. They insist on adding sugar where it has no place being.

Dr. Lustig uses yogurt and chocolate milk as examples of unnecessary added sugars.

Comparing a 20-ounce Coca-Cola with a 6-ounce Yoplait yogurt, we find they both contain 27 grams of "total sugars". If the sugar in the "healthy" yogurt was lactose that would be fine, but it's not. Only 16 grams is natural lactose, they added another 11 grams of sucrose. That's like eating the yogurt and drinking an 8-ounce Coke.

Same deal with another dairy favorite, chocolate milk. An 8-ounce carton of one percent milk has 130 calories and 15 grams of "total sugars" (lactose). However, an 8-ounce carton of one percent chocolate milk has 190 calories and 29 grams of "total sugars," including 14 grams of added sugar (HFCS). So chocolate milk is milk plus 10 ounces of Coca-Cola.

[29]Ethanol - Alcohol

This is a book about sugar but there are other ways of getting fat. It's only fair that we mention how alcohol is metabolized so you can compare the damage from a giant soda to that of a stiff drink.

---

27   http://en.wikipedia.org/wiki/Galactose
28   http://en.wikipedia.org/wiki/Lactase
29   http://en.wikipedia.org/wiki/Ethanol

Studies of alcohol use show that a little bit is good for us. Alcohol raises HDL (good cholesterol), and red wine has the compound resveratrol, which is thought to improve insulin sensitivity and longevity. But more than a glass or two a day is a very different story.

When carbohydrates are fermented a by-product called ethanol is produced.

To use our example of 120 calories, we can drink 1½ ounces of 80 proof liquor. 10% of the 120 calories (12) is metabolized in the stomach and intestines. A further 10% is metabolized in the brain, which is what gets us intoxicated. The remaining 96 calories go to the liver. That's 24 more calories than from sucrose (glucose/fructose). But, just like fructose, the ethanol goes directly to the mitochondria instead of being turned into glycogen which is what happens to glucose.

Then, of course, there are all the additional problems caused by excess alcohol consumption such as alcoholic liver disease, liver insulin resistance and death.

Life runs on chemistry. There are no levers, switches or gears. No hard drives, LEDs or circuit boards. Even the software that runs everything is chemically based. The ones and zeros of our digital computers are replaced with guanine, adenine, thymine, and cytosine, the G, A, T, C of the DNA molecule[30].

The processes that break down our food into usable energy are no different, it's all run by chemical messages. Chemicals that make us hungry, chemicals that tell us we're full and chemicals that tell our body to store extra energy as fat.

Millions of evolutionary years designed these systems. It has only taken thirty years or so for the Evil Empire to screw it up, leading to the reasons we are all getting fat.

METABOLIC CHEMICAL MESSENGERS

Our body is pre-programmed to release specific hormones under certain conditions and it is also pre-programmed to react to those hormones in specific ways. Each of these reactions have been programmed into our DNA over millions of years of evolution.

This is the first time in the history of the human race that food has been plentiful for almost everyone. Before now, the best survival tactic had been to store food while it was plentiful in expectation that a period of famine was coming,

The problem now is that there is no famine in the western world and, worse still, the Evil Empire is deliberately manipulating our most basic reactions in order to sell more and more of their food-like products.

There are dozens of different chemicals involved in the metabolic process but they are really only of interest to the scientists that study the causes of obesity. For our purposes, we only need to focus on seven hormones and how our food turns into belly fat.

---

30   http://en.wikipedia.org/wiki/DNA

Our body is at work 24/7 so all the processes are ongoing. We have to choose an arbitrary point in the eating cycle to explain how the process works.

[31]Hypothalamus

The hypothalamus is part of the limbic system which includes the hippocampus, amygdala and thalamus. It's a small area (about one cubic centimeter) of the brain, located just below the thalamus, that automatically controls a lot of the body's systems like temperature, circadian rhythm, hunger and thirst. It responds to chemical triggers that it receives via the bloodstream.

[32]Ghrelin

The eating cycle begins with the peptide ghrelin. When the body clicks over to starvation mode our stomach starts to produce ghrelin. The longer we go without eating the more ghrelin that gets produced.

The hypothalamus interprets the presence of this hormone in the bloodstream as hunger and we get the urge to eat.

As our stomach fills, the production of ghrelin goes down but that is not what stops us from eating, that's the job of PYY which we will get to in a minute.

Fructose does not affect the production of ghrelin. This means the super-sized soda we drink before a meal adds an enormous calorie hit without contributing to our satiety.

It has also been shown that stress will prompt the body to produce ghrelin, so score another hit for the Evil Empire. Job security, medical bills, housing crisis, terrorist threats, the government and Wall Street branches of the Evil Empire can take some of the blame for our obesity because their actions make us hungry.

---

31   http://en.wikipedia.org/wiki/Hypothalamus
32   http://en.wikipedia.org/wiki/Ghrelin

[33]Dopamine

Dopamine is chemical pleasure. More precisely, it's a neurotransmitter that activates the pleasure centers of our brains. When dopamine is released our brains say, "Oh, that's good".

When we start to eat, dopamine is released and, as a reward for eating, we feel pleasure. As long as dopamine is being produced we will continue to eat. When the dopamine is suppressed we stop eating because our brain decides we have had enough.

Sometimes the system can get out of whack and the dopamine receptors get desensitized. When that happens, it takes more dopamine to have the same effect.

Drug addicts often experience this resistance effect and end up taking more and more of their drug of choice to get the same high, (see the addiction section below).

[34]Leptin

Leptin is an incredibly important hormone that nobody knew about until 1994. It is produced by fat tissue and informs the hypothalamus that we have eaten enough.

The amount of leptin in our system is directly proportional to the amount of body fat we carry. Our body will do all it can to maintain this relationship which is what makes dieting so difficult.

As the amount of fat tissue goes down so does the amount of leptin which triggers our bodies to enter starvation mode. In turn, that makes us eat more and reduce activity. This is not a fast acting strategy but more of a transitional switch from times of famine to times of plenty.

Adequate levels of leptin help suppress the production of dopamine which means we are no longer being rewarded for eating. But if we are leptin resistant, the dopamine production does not get suppressed and we continue to eat. (see below)

---

33   http://en.wikipedia.org/wiki/Dopamine
34   http://en.wikipedia.org/wiki/Leptin

Another problem comes from high insulin levels which block the action of leptin on the hypothalamus and make the hypothalamus think we're staving, causing us to eat more.

[35]Insulin

The liver releases glucose into the circulatory system and it is taken up by the cells in our body and used as energy. Any excess glucose will find its way to our pancreas and causes the pancreas to produce insulin.

When the system is in balance, the pancreas releases just enough insulin to store the excess glucose as fat. It opens our fat cells and stuffs the glucose into them by converting the glucose to triglycerides.

Insulin also has the job of clearing dopamine from the synapses which means, as our insulin levels increase, the pleasure we get from eating is reduced and we put our fork down.

When insulin levels drop the body shifts into reverse and starts burning those stored triglycerides. The fat cells shrink, the fat enters the bloodstream and travels back to the liver where it is converted back to chemical energy.

The result - we lose weight.

Insulin makes fat. Without it your fat cells stay empty.

[36]Glycogen

Glycogen, (liver starch) is a form of glucose that our liver stores as a source of quick energy. Glycogen is good. It is our body's preferred method to store excess energy. When quick energy is needed, stored glycogen is converted back to glucose so it can be used throughout the body.

The conversion of glucose to glycogen is controlled by insulin but sometimes excess glucose gets stored as fat, which we don't want.

While total glycogen depletion is rare for most of us, endurance athletes, such as marathon runners, cross country skiers and long-distance cyclers may experience this type of depletion if they do not make attempts to

35   http://en.wikipedia.org/wiki/Insulin
36   http://en.wikipedia.org/wiki/Glycogen

restore their glycogen levels. We've all heard the term "hitting the wall" in conjunction with such endurance sports. This usually refers to such a depletion of glycogen and the athlete simply has no energy stores left and cannot continue.

[37]PYY - Peptide YY(3-36)

Known as the satiety hormone, PYY is ultimately what stops us from eating. This peptide is released into the bloodstream when food reaches the end of twenty-two feet of small intestine.

Clearly, if we want to eat less, we need to do all we can to speed our food through the small intestine. The best way to do that is to include a lot of fiber with our meal. That means staying away from processed food because most of the fiber has been removed to either improve taste or shelf life, or both.

We also need to allow time for this process to work. The best way to help this process work properly is to slow down our eating and wait at least twenty minutes before we have a second helping or a sugary dessert.

[38]Cortisol

Cortisol is the stress hormone. The adrenal gland (on top of our kidneys) releases cortisol into the blood stream whenever we are being chased by a ferocious wild animal. At least, that is what evolution designed it to do.

When cortisol enters our bloodstream it raises blood pressure, increases blood glucose levels and increases our heart rate. All good stuff when we're running for our lives. In this kind of life-or-death situation, we either get away and can relax or we get eaten and our hormone levels simply don't matter anymore.

We can't survive without cortisol. There's always a certain level in our system to affect and control a variety of processes. In this book, we are only concerned with the roll it plays in insulin resistance, obesity and metabolic syndrome.

37   http://en.wikipedia.org/wiki/Peptide_YY
38   http://en.wikipedia.org/wiki/Cortisol

The descriptions of the processes influenced by cortisol, and the effects of continued high levels, are beyond the purview of this book. However, Dr. Lustig devotes chapter 6 of his book, "Fat Chance", to a detailed explanation.

He shows how high cortisol levels cause us to eat more which leads to weight gain. He also shows that the lower we are on the social economic scale the higher our level of stress and the more likely we are to be overweight due to high cortisol levels.

It's no surprise that the US population is getting so fat when a huge percentage is under almost constant stress. No social safety net, right to work states and, until recently, no health care.

Over the past thirty years, the income gap between the middle class and the top one percent of income earners has been steadily widening. Compare the progress of this gap on a graph with the increase in obesity and metabolic syndrome and they match perfectly.

[39] Triglycerides

Triglycerides are the main component of vegetable oils and animal fat. In the context of this book we are referring to the fat that floats in our bloodstreams and eventually gets deposited around the organs in the abdomen.

---

39   http://en.wikipedia.org/wiki/Triglyceride

Leptin Resistance

As we said earlier, leptin was only discovered in 1994 so much of the work to decipher exactly all the roles it plays in our bodies is ongoing.

Some things that are known include the fact that the more fat we carry the higher our leptin levels are.

Various studies have shown that fructose is a major cause of leptin resistance.

Leptin resistance is a condition where, for some reason, our hypothalamus does not adequately react to the leptin in our blood. Our brain believes we are starving and increases our energy storage (fat deposits) and conserves energy (lethargy).

COUNTERACTING LEPTIN RESISTANCE

This is currently an area of intense research and there are no conclusive answers. Most studies seem to indicate that regular exercise is an important factor along with specific dietary recommendations. Our best advice is to search the Internet for the latest research. But be warned, this is a hot topic and the trolls will be out in force trying to sell their snake oil and magic beans.

Insulin Resistance

Insulin controls the primary functions of our appetite. When it's low we burn the stored triglycerides around our waist. As our insulin levels rise the pleasurable effects of dopamine are reduced and we stop eating.

INSULIN RESISTANCE

[40]Insulin resistance is what happens when cells become less responsive to the controlling effects of insulin. Insulin resistant liver cells result in less production of glycogen and storage of excess glucose. The liver continues to produce glucose.

Insulin resistance can occur in a variety of cells and refers to the cells ability to respond correctly to the presence of insulin.

Fatty liver is not responsive to insulin so the pancreas has to make more insulin to overcome the resistance of the liver to do its job.

CAUSE OF INSULIN RESISTANCE

The exact cause of insulin resistance is not completely understood but various studies have found that the major contributors to the condition are high fat diets and fructose. High amounts of visceral fat have been shown to cause insulin resistance, which in turn promotes diabetes, cancer, cardiovascular disease, dementia, and aging.

SIGNS OF INSULIN RESISTANCE

Although it is not very scientific, a good indicator that you may be insulin resistent is your waist measurement. If you are male and your waist measurement is more than 40 inches (101 cm) or if you are female and your waist measurement is more than 35 inches (89 cm), you are carrying too much visceral fat and are a candidate for insulin resistance.

---

40   http://en.wikipedia.org/wiki/Insulin_resistance

It's In Our DNA

How did we evolve to get fat? What was happening to our ancestors that made fat a survival trait that should be passed on to future generations?

Before our supermarkets were stocked with every conceivable food, year round, there was something called seasons. Most fruits used to appear in the fall - just before winter when very little fresh food is available.

It made sense for our forebears to binge on the available fruit and put down a layer of visceral fat that would help them to get through the months of winter famine. This is a strategy still followed by many wild animals today.

Effects of Insulin Resistance

Since insulin is one of our primary hormones, if our bodies do not respond correctly insulin resistance causes many problems. Our biological systems are controlled by chemical messengers, so insulin resistance is equivalent to throwing a giant wrench (spanner) in the works of a mechanical system.

As the problem gets steadily worse the pancreas can't keep up with the demands of producing more and more insulin. When this happens, we call it type 2 diabetes. If you're lucky you can control it by going on the kind of diet you should be on in the first place. If not, you must inject yourself with insulin made in a lab.

Insulin is a hormone that plays a part in cell division and cancer is, essentially, a problem of uncontrolled cell division. It's called hyperinsulinemia and is associated with the development and growth of various forms of cancer.

Insulin resistance is also suspected as a possible cause of dementia.

Women not only get all of the above but insulin resistance can cause their ovaries to make extra testosterone and less estrogen. If they carry particular genes, this can results in [41]polycystic ovarian syndrome, hirsutism (excess body hair), and infertility.

---

41   http://en.wikipedia.org/wiki/Polycystic_ovary_syndrome

INSULIN RESISTANCE TREATMENT

Treating insulin resistance, also called pre-diabetes, is a lot easier than dealing with full blown type 2 diabetes.

All we have to do is give the Evil Empire the finger. Simply change our diet to eliminate processed foods, stop smoking, get moderate exercise and proper sleep.

That may sound glib and self serving given the title of this book but it is absolutely true. It is time for us to realize that the big food companies are poisoning the population for profit.

Be sure to read Section 4 Corporate Complicity to find out about all the dirty tricks these bottom feeders get up to and about how a government that is supposed to protect us turns a blind eye in return for campaign donations.

[42]Dietary Fiber

For some reason, we have come to think of fiber as a waste product of food. If we think of it at all, it's as a pill or drink we take when we're constipated.

We didn't evolve that way. Our ancient ancestors ate 100 grams of fiber a day. Now, the average person eats only 12 grams per day. It's the fiber content in fruit that protects us from the fructose. In the name of progress we have removed most, or all, of the fiber from fruit juices and packaged foods so they will keep longer. The trouble is, without the fiber, the fructose not only goes directly to fat, it creates a greater load for our liver to deal with.

The fiber eaten with a meal turns into a gelatinous barrier between the wall of the intestine and the digesting food. This barrier delays the absorption of glucose, fructose and fat.

If the pancreas doesn't sense a sharp rise in blood glucose it responds by producing less insulin. Less insulin means less glucose gets pushed into the fat cells.

Type 2 diabetics can potentially reduce their blood sugar levels by a third if they switch to a high fiber diet.

Fiber helps to keep food moving through the intestines. Without it our internal food processing system backs up, the food in our gut putrefies and we end up with colon cancer.

There are two kinds of fiber in the food we eat - soluble and insoluble. What does that mean?

[43]Insoluble Fiber

Insoluble fiber is great for moving things along through your gut and colon. Because this kind of fiber doesn't dissolve in water, it remains virtually intact as it passes through us. That speeds food and waste through our system and helps to prevent constipation.

---

42   http://en.wikipedia.org/wiki/Dietary_fiber
43   http://www.webmd.com/diet/fiber-health-benefits-11/insoluble-soluble-fiber

Some good sources of insoluble fiber are: whole grains, nuts, celery, broccoli, cabbage, dark leafy greens, raisins (and grapes), several root vegetables (with the skins left on), barley, whole kernel corn.

Soluble Fiber

Soluble fiber can actually slow down the digestion process. But that's not a bad thing. The soluble types of fiber combine with water to form a gel. It helps to delay the emptying of our stomach, making us feel full. This can have a positive effect by helping to keep blood sugar at normal levels and by reducing insulin sensitivity. It may even help lower the bad LDL associated with cholesterol.

Some good sources of soluble fiber are: oatmeal, lentils, apples, oat bran, flaxseeds (ground), blueberries, cucumbers and carrots.

Some of these fruits and vegetables contain both soluble and insoluble fiber.

How Much Dietary Fiber Do We Need?

The short answer is as much as we can get. It is unlikely that any modern diet is going to contain more dietary fiber than we can handle.

Our perfectly evolved ancestors consumed around 100 grams of fiber a day, whereas our peers today only eat an average of 12 grams. The recommended daily allowance is double the average at 25 grams but when it comes to fiber more is definitely better.

How Does Fiber Affect Fructose?

As noted above, the fiber barrier delays the absorption of fructose which gives our liver a chance to deal with it. The liver changes the fructose to acetyl-CoA which is burned in the mitochondrial Krebs cycle, but that is beyond the scope of this book.

Does A High Fiber Diet Help Us Lose Weight?

Not directly. Adding fiber to a diet and keeping the calorie intake the same won't make any difference. But, by eating a high fiber diet we will most likely eat less. High fiber foods tend to be less calorie dense so we will eat fewer calories for the same amount of food.

Also we need to chew foods that contain a high amount of fiber. That means we eat more slowly which gives our body the chance to send satiety signals to our brain.

How Do We Get More Fiber?

Stay away from packaged and "fast" foods. Most of the fiber has been removed to improve shelf life. Eat fresh, whole foods.

What Is Fat?

When we step on the scales we are weighing our entire body; bones, muscle, subcutaneous fat and visceral fat. We don't want to lose any weight from our bones. We want good, strong, dense bones, particularly as we get older.

We want more muscle tissue, too, not less, because it is the mitochondria in our muscles that burns the glucose. As we increase muscle our body becomes more sensitive to insulin and our health improves regardless of our overall weight.

[44]Subcutaneous Fat

This is the layer of fat just below our skin. It provides padding, insulation and energy stores.

Subcutaneous fat, also called adipose tissue, accounts for about 80% of our total body fat. Up to a point, this is good fat. Studies have shown a correlation between longevity and the amount of subcutaneous fat we carry.

[45]White Fat

Adipose tissue comes in two types, white fat (WAT) and brown fat (BAT).

If we are healthy and not overweight our white fat accounts for 20% of our body weight if we're male and 25% if female.

White fat responds to insulin, growth hormones [46]norepinephrine (which releases energy in the [47]flight or fight response) and [48]glucocorticoids (to stimulate fat breakdown).

White fat is the primary source of leptin. Although 20 - 25% for males and females is a good percentage, any greater and leptin levels would be too high and could lead to leptin resistance.

---

44   http://en.wikipedia.org/wiki/Subcutaneous_tissue
45   http://en.wikipedia.org/wiki/White_adipose_tissue
46   http://en.wikipedia.org/wiki/Norepinephrine
47   http://en.wikipedia.org/wiki/Fight-or-flight_response
48   http://en.wikipedia.org/wiki/Glucocorticoid

[49]Brown Fat

Brown fat generates heat and is especially abundant in newborns. In adult humans it is still present in the upper chest and neck.

The brown color is caused by a high number of iron-containing mitochondria. The mitochondria burn excess glucose which, of course, is a good thing. We want all the brown fat we can get to help with weight loss.

In a study recently published by [50]The Journal of Clinical Investigation researchers showed that obesity causes brown fat to whiten. This potentially leads to a spiral effect of greater obesity and less brown fat until all the brown fat has whitened.

[51]Irisin - (Fibronectin domain-containing protein 5)

Irisin is a peptide hormone that our bodies produce when we exercise. It was identified in 2002 but it was only in 2012 that a study using mice identified some potential health benefits for humans.

The results are not yet confirmed but irisin has the potential of generating weight loss and blocking diabetes.

Several independent studies confirm that irisin appears to convert white fat to healthy brown fat. We recommend reading a report on the subject published in Disease Models and Mechanisms. It's very technical but if you can get past all the stuff that's unpronounceable it's very interesting.

http://dmm.biologists.org/content/5/3/293.full?sid=3af43439-5966-4ee6-92b0-e66e2a4593a5

Essentially, it says that endurance exercise will turn white fat into brown fat and help with metabolic syndrome. How effective this is for humans is still not clear but this is certainly something that bears watching.

---

49   http://en.wikipedia.org/wiki/Brown_adipose_tissue
50   http://www.jci.org/articles/view/71643
51   http://en.wikipedia.org/wiki/FNDC5

[52]*Visceral Fat*

Around 20% of our total body fat, or 4 to 6 percent of our total body weight, is visceral fat. That roll of fat around our belly is visceral fat. It's in our liver and around our organs. This is the bad stuff. This is the fat that will kill us.

The good news is that visceral fat is the first to be burned and will disappear first once we eliminate fructose from our diet, exercise regularly and get our metabolic hormones in balance.

Visceral fat is made up of triglycerides which is the body's way of transferring extra energy.

Visceral fat is the whole crux of the obesity epidemic. People will always come in various sizes - fat, thin and just right - but without that spare tire we stand to get an extra 15 years of life.

Carrying that extra belly fat can mean insulin resistance, diabetes, cancer, cardiovascular disease, dementia and premature aging. Is it worth it?

[53]*Triglycerides*

Triglycerides stored in our muscles and as belly fat were good for our primitive ancestors because it was a source of quick energy. When we were being chased by something with big teeth we certainly wanted to get super charged fast.

Nowadays, we don't encounter a whole lot of man eating ferocious beasts on Main Street so our belly just sort of hangs there and blocks the view of our feet.

---

52   http://en.wikipedia.org/wiki/Adipose_tissue
53   http://www.heart.org/HEARTORG/GettingHealthy/ NutritionCenter/Triglycerides_UCM_306029_Article.jsp

Obesity & Metabolic-Syndrome

There's a lot of buzz lately about "Metabolic Syndrome". Most people have heard about it but few understand what it is.

Metabolic syndrome is not a disease, it's a collection of diseases with a common cause. It is associated with obesity because roughly 80% of obese people have one or more of these conditions. But being obese does not mean we will suffer from one of these conditions, only that we are more likely to. And, even if someone is not obese, that doesn't mean they can't fall victim to these conditions. After all, up to 40 percent of normal-weight adults have one or more of these conditions.

When we do a little math with these percentages we discover that there are many more normal weight people with these conditions than obese people, simply because 70% of the population is normal weight.

◊ Type 2 diabetes

◊ Hypertension (high blood pressure)

◊ Heart (cardiovascular) disease

◊ Lipid (blood fat) disorders

◊ Cancer

◊ Dementia

The important take away from this is that it is metabolic syndrome that will kill us - not obesity. The other important point is that insulin resistance is the common factor among metabolic syndrome patients, not obesity.

One of the most disturbing facts to surface recently is that, for the first time in history, our children have a shorter life expectancy than their parents.

When the liver is overwhelmed by foodstuffs that cannot be metabolized by other organs, or by the mitochondria in our cells, it can lead to metabolic syndrome. Fructose can only be metabolized by the liver so an excess of fructose goes directly to fat.

The Exercise Factor

Our body is very efficient and it can do a lot with a small amount of energy. For example, a can of Coke will provide all the energy we need to play badminton for 24 minutes, take a 30 minute walk, cycle for 36 minutes, garden for 32 minutes and more.

Coca Cola in the UK provides a resource site for these kinds of calculations. http://www.coca-cola.co.uk/health/work-it-out-calculator.html#

Keep in mind, though, that Coke in the UK does NOT have HFCS in it - only sugar. Still bad for us but not as bad as Coke purchased in the US. But the calculator they provide could be a valuable visual reference for how long exercise actually takes to burn off any significant quantities of calories

However, this simple comparison shows us that if we think we can eat all we want and just exercise it off - forget about it. It's not going to happen. Exercise as a calorie burning plan is a bad idea.

But we can't let that deter us from getting regular exercise. Even a modest amount of exercise is essential to any weight loss plan, or at least to any plan to get healthy. Weight loss is a secondary consideration to achieving good health.

Why do we need to exercise? Because exercise builds muscle.

Why do we need more muscle? Because muscle tissue contains the mitochondria that burns the glucose as fuel.

Why does exercise alone not lead to significant weight loss? Because we're building muscle and muscle weighs more than fat.

Want more reasons to exercise? Exercise releases endorphins.

Feeling blue? Have some aches and pains? Try going for a walk.

The key, however, is to maintain a regular exercise regimen. And by that, we don't mean that we have to do a strenuous work out every day. However, we do need to move our body, if not every day, every couple of days.

With our busy lives we can hear a lot of people saying, "But I just don't have the time." Are we really trying to say that we can't go for a 15 minute walk every couple of days? Is our health not worth even that little bit of time? And, with the advent of some interactive video games, we can even get some of our exercise indoors during cold or inclement weather.

We have great fun playing bowling and tennis, along with other physical-type video games, on our game console. And don't try to tell us it's not "real" exercise. We really overdid it one day and had the muscle aches to prove it!

We don't need to join a gym, buy exercise or jogging clothes, drag ourselves out of the house at dawn each day to bicycle around our neighborhood. All we need to do is commit to moving our body on a regular basis. Walking and swimming are both great exercises, so if joining a gym is part of the plan, try to find one with a pool and/or a jogging/walking track.

Toning our muscles means they will burn more calories and those muscles will not only thank us but reward us, too. We'll feel better. We may even feel great! Where's the downside?

When Do Calories Count?

We have learned that not all calories are equal. There are good calories and there are bad calories but the laws of thermodynamics still apply. If we consume more than we burn the excess will be stored as fat. That will never change. The trick is to only consume calories that are easily burned and not the ones that go directly to fat in our liver.

We must also be mindful of the extra calories we can consume without it having any effect on our satiety. Dropping into 7-Eleven for a [54]44 ounce Super Big Gulp will add 512 calories to our day without any significant reduction in our ghrelin levels. Think of it this way - would we want to consume 128 grams of sugar, (32 teaspoons) by the spoonful? Because that's how much sugar we're getting without feeling full at all.

Later in the day if we stopped by McDonald's for a 22 ounce McCafé Chocolate Shake we would add another 850 calories. That's another 120 grams (30 teaspoons) of sugar.

Maybe tomorrow we'd be tempted to try a 64 ounce Pepsi at KFC. That's 780 calories from 217 grams of sugar (54 teaspoons). Remember half of those calories come from fructose which goes directly to fat.

Daily Allowance

The percentage of daily allowance figures on food labels are based on a 2000 calorie a day diet which is what a hypothetical average person will burn in a day. Our [55]height, weight, sex and activity level will change these estimates. We must keep our caloric intake below our personal daily allowance if we want to lose weight.

So the first rule is: DON'T DRINK YOUR CALORIES!

---

54   http://www.sugarstacks.com/beverages.htm
55   http://www.hikingupward.com/cal_calc.asp

Overweight and Healthy,
Skinny and Sick

Some people just eat too much, are overweight, but are otherwise perfectly healthy. There are also people that live on sugary drinks and cookies and are skinny but very, very sick.

Calories count but some calories do a lot more harm than others.

By reviewing what we said at the beginning about our bodies being run by chemicals, we can understand why an upset in the chemical balance can have disastrous effects on our weight. We can have all the will power in the world but if our body's basic systems are screaming "I'm starving", we don't stand a chance.

This is not to say we should just throw our hands in the air and say, "I give". We now know what the problems are so we know enough to stop drinking our calories. We also know not to eat packaged and processed foods.

Combine that knowledge with a little bit of regular exercise and we can give the Evil Empire the finger.

Bottom Line On Obesity Management

Diets don't work. That's hardly news to anyone that's spent a lifetime trying to lose weight. Our leptin levels want to remain at the current set point and will fight us all the way unless we can reset the levels. We can't fight our hormones, we have to correct the balance between them.

Following these steps will help:
1. To reduce our insulin levels - cut out all processed food, carbonated drinks and fruit juice. This will reduce body fat and improve leptin resistance.

2. To reduce our body's level of ghrelin - eat a large protein breakfast as soon as we get up in the morning. This way our body won't produce the ghrelin that makes us feel hungry.

3. Eat lots of fiber - a diet high in soluble and insoluble fiber will slow digestion and speed food through the intestine to quickly raise our level of PYY which tells our hypothalamus that we should stop eating.

4. Don't sweat the small stuff - stress increases cortisol levels and cortisol makes us eat more. Get lots of sleep and do yoga or whatever it takes to reduce stress levels.

5. Take time to exercise - lots of good things happen with even moderate exercise - we eat less, feel better and make brown fat.

Section 3 Sugar Addiction

Can sugar actually be as addictive, or even more addictive, than cocaine? It appears so. In a 2007 study conducted by scientists Magalie Lenoir, Fuschia Serre, Lauriane Cantin and Serge H. Ahmed, 94% of rats that were allowed to chose between cocaine and refined sugar, chose sugar. That even included rats that were previously addicted to cocaine and changed their preference to sugar.

Sugar Addiction

WHY SUGAR IS ADDICTIVE
The Evolution Factor

It took millions of years for us to evolve to the point where we were perfectly adapted to our environment. Now we have changed our environment and, by doing that, it appears that we are no longer able to evolve through the process of natural selection.

Our best survival adaptation for today is a willingness to go against the crowd, the ability to just say no. Don't believe the advertisements and lies. Stand up and say this is wrong and refuse to be a lab rat.

We originally evolved to seek out tastes that are sweet, salty and fatty in order to survive. Young children are particularly predisposed to crave these kinds of tastes as a survival tactic to ensure that they eat sufficient calories. Developing such preferences meant that our children would take in sufficient calories to be able to survive into adulthood.

Receiving a pleasurable reward (endorphins) for eating helped to ensure the survival of our species. However, we developed this survival technique when sweet-tasting foods were not easily available. In today's world we have easy access to an overabundance of sugary products. We no longer have to expend an enormous number of calories in order to obtain high calorie foods.

In most cases, sugar now comes packaged with fat and salt, a combination that we find irresistible. After all, who doesn't like cake, pie, cookies, etc. But there is a lot of "hidden" sugar in packaged and highly processed foods, sometimes even in totally unexpected places - like our toothpaste!

HOW WE GET ADDICTED TO SUGAR

According to Michael Moss' best selling book *Salt Sugar Fat: How the Food Giants Hooked Us*, the food companies know exactly what they are doing and spend copious amounts of money on research in order to formulate their recipes to invoke our "bliss point", the point where there is exactly the right amount of sugar and/or fat and/or salt to send our taste buds and our senses into absolute bliss, knowingly hooking us in order to keep us coming back for more.

Now, doesn't this seem like the same kind of behavior the tobacco companies used (and got caught doing) when they added more nicotine to cigarettes to get their customers hooked? Well, guess what - a lot of the tobacco companies now own the food companies. Do we honestly believe that they would abandon such tactics just because they're now in the food industry?

According to [1]LiveScience, "*A major hallmark of addiction is a loss of control regarding use of a substance — such as taking more than you should, or escalating your use despite knowing the substance is harmful — as well as cravings for it.*"

That sure sounds like sugar to us.

NEEDING MORE TO GET SAME "BUZZ"

We have become sensitized to the amount of sugar we consume because of the quantities involved. In essence, what that means is, we need more of the stuff to get the same impact - put more clearly - we need more and more just to get the same buzz, just like any other addictive drug.

We have all noticed it - the more sugar we have, the more we crave. But it's gradual and often we don't even realize it until we STOP consuming sugar. When we make a concerted effort to eliminate sugar from our food, we find that things we used to enjoy, like the occasional chocolate bar, now seem sickeningly sweet. Really! Try it.

When we consciously kick the sugar habit we will be able to enjoy the natural sweetness of foods that, because of our overconsumption of sugar, may have seemed bland to us.

KICKING THE HABIT

Like any addiction, kicking the habit is not easy. However, kicking our sugar habit, given its ubiquitous presence in our food supply, can seem nearly impossible. Many of us are consuming sugar, in startlingly large amounts, without actually being aware of it.

---

1   http://www.livescience.com/40749-addiction-drugs-sugar.html

Our first step to kicking the habit is being able to identify all the added sugar that food manufactures try to sneak by us by using other names for it. (See Other Names of Sugar)

Too often, when we decide we need to eliminate sugar and lose weight, we start to feel like we're depriving ourselves, denying ourselves a means to experience pleasure. It's a common response.

Feeling this way creates stress, stress activates cortisol and, you guessed it, we eat more of the things we shouldn't and gain more belly fat. When we feel stressed our body craves high calorie foods loaded with sugar.

We need to convince ourselves that healthy alterations to the way we eat are not only going to provide us with those pleasure signals but also ensure that we will remain healthy and fit.

Yes, we've all said it (or at least thought it), "Poor me, I can't have that donut because I'm on a diet." What we should really be saying is, "I won't have that donut because it is full of sugar, fat, processed flour and it is POISON!" Should we really feel bad about not putting poison into our body? Of course not.

Okay, yes, we do know that maintaining that kind of mind-set can be difficult. We're the first to admit that we still often crave those high sugar, high fat, highly processed foods. It's tough, but not impossible, to train yourself to WANT to avoid such things.

Case in point: We had a tradition when we went on road trips. During our stops, either for a break or to fill up with gas, we liked to grab either a couple of donuts or a couple of candy bars.

On one of our more recent road trips, we bought the requisite candy bars while filling up with gas. We both looked forward to eating them, we may have even begun salivating. When we took the first few bites we discovered something amazing - we both found the candy bars way too sweet, much sweeter than we had remembered.

The only thing we could put this down to was that, for many weeks before this particular road trip, we had significantly reduced our sugar intake from both self-added (sugar in coffee, sugar on cereal, etc.) and hidden (check the ingredients on any packaged or process foods, like spaghetti sauce, peanut butter, salad dressing, etc. for the many different names) sugar.

We did finish the candy bars. Yes, we know we should have just thrown them away, after all, they're poison, right? Yes, that's right, but we are far too frugal for our own good and simply could not accept wasting something we had paid for.

However, it taught us a valuable lesson. Now, when we THINK we are craving a candy bar, particularly on a road trip, we can remind ourselves that we not only know it's poison but that we will find it disgustingly sweet. The cravings are still there and that little devil on our shoulder keeps trying to convince us that this time it will be different, this time we really want that candy bar. So far we've been able to resist the temptation but it often takes some real convincing.

WITHDRAWAL SYMPTOMS

According to [2]LiveStrong, the most common symptom of sugar withdrawal is headaches. These should be temporary as our body adjusts to a sugar-free diet.

However, other symptoms are also possible and these can include fatigue, tremors, depression and anxiety. That's right - just like withdrawing from an addictive drug.

While the length of withdrawal will vary from person to person, usually the symptoms will only last for a few days.

THE DOSE MAKES THE POISON

The term "the dose makes the poison" is most often credited to [3]Paracelsus, as Swiss-German physician born in 1493.

---

2   http://www.livestrong.com/article/309515-can-cutting-sugar-out-of-a-diet-cause-headaches/
3   http://en.wikipedia.org/wiki/Paracelsus

ACUTE POISON VS CHRONIC POISON

Not only is sugar addictive, it is also a toxin. That's right, it's a poison! However, it is a chronic poison that takes its toll in small increments.

An acute poison is something that will, potentially, kill us almost immediately - like cyanide.

A chronic poison is something that will take a long time to kill us but, make no mistake, it will kill us. Sugar is just such a poison.

It's unfortunate that the rush of pleasure we receive when consuming high-sugar foods may dilute our resolve to avoid this chronic poison. After all, our predisposition to sweet tastes was originally a survival tactic.

In the wild, poisons are usually bitter and a sweet taste generally means that something is safe to eat. Honey is a good example. It is the only food that doesn't go bad and supplies nutrients as well. It is also naturally anti-bacterial and was often used to treat wounds. Is it any wonder that we developed the belief that sweet tasting foods equal not only good, but safe?

However, now that we control our environment, rather than evolving to exist with our environment, our bodies have not been able to make the switch to lessen our cravings for sweet - not to mention fats and salt. And, the recent addition of High Fructose Corn Syrup to a huge number of packaged/prepared foods just makes it that much more difficult.

As we learned earlier, Fructose is not metabolized by the body the same way that glucose is. We NEED glucose, it is used by every cell in our body. Fructose, on the other hand, puts a heavy burden on our liver and increases our belly fat - all while tasting very, very good. It's like we just can't catch a break.

RISE IN CHRONIC DISEASES

Our addiction to sugar appears to be tied to the rise in several chronic diseases, with type 2 diabetes leading the way. Doesn't it make sense that a chronic poison would result in chronic diseases?

There have been many studies that support this claim and the incidences of these chronic diseases rise right alongside the increase in sugar consumption.

As we said, right at the beginning, we are not scientists, but we can read, we can research, we can think. And, some of this information just seems so obvious to us.

It's no secret that refined sugars, and particularly High Fructose Corn Syrup, are bad for us. Why then is there any resistance to the idea that these refined sugars, being consumed in enormous amounts, cause chronic diseases?

It just follows that if we knowingly consume something that is an obvious poison that we will, naturally, suffer the consequences.

That is another hallmark of an addiction - even though we KNOW it is bad for us, we continue to use it.

Sugar - A Substitute For Happiness?

Yet another way we can become addicted to sugar is by using it, many times unknowingly, as a substitute for happiness. This can happen when we confuse pleasure for happiness.

We've all turned to food when we're upset, unhappy or depressed. Why? Because food gives us pleasure and pleasure can be a short term replacement for happiness. It's easy to confuse the two.

Feeling pleasure makes us feel happy most of the time, but it is a temporary thing and when the pleasure recedes then we can become unhappy. That starts the vicious cycle of using food as a means to feel pleasure but each low afterwards drives us to eat more in order to experience the pleasure again and the cycle continues.

More often than not, when we seek pleasure from food, particularly when we are feeling low, we seek out high-sugar, high-carb and high-fat foods because they can quickly deliver that rush of pleasure and give us an immediate boost. However, after the initial rush comes the crash. We've all experienced the sugar high followed by the sugar low. And when the crash happens, we feel even worse than we did when we turned to food to lift our mood in the first place.

This, naturally, leads to more cravings for high-sugar foods to regain the feeling of pleasure. As this cycle continues, according to Dr. Robert Lustig, your pleasure receptors down-regulate, meaning more sugar is needed to achieve the same level of pleasure.

Why Does This Happen?

With excessive sugar intake comes insulin resistance. We then also become leptin resistant and we are unable to clear the dopamine from our pleasure receptors. That means that we just keep getting rewarded for eating, so we keep eating. The leptin isn't able to remove the dopamine reward so we're not able to get the signal to stop eating. We think we're still hungry, that's the signals we're getting and, in addition, we keep getting rewarded for eating.

Vicious Cycle

As we said, it's a vicious cycle and it can be very difficult to break. However, we need to because these highs and lows are very hard on our system.

In order to break the cycle, just like with any addictive substance, we will have to go through the withdrawal symptoms, which are unique to each of us. Some of us will, for the most part, breeze through the withdrawal, but some of us will have to work much harder to break the cycle and will suffer more extreme effects from the withdrawal.

The good news is, we CAN break the cycle and stop putting this chronic poison into our bodies.

Don't Be Held Hostage By The Evil Empire

If we allow our sugar addiction to continue, then the Evil Empire wins. They get to continue peddling their poison.

These huge corporations don't care about our health, all they care about is their bottom line and getting us hooked means that they have a steady stream of income.

The only way to stop the Evil Empire is to hit them where it hurts - their income.

Voting with our dollars has been very effective in the past and it can be just as effective now. Refuse to support them - don't buy their poison. It's the only way to get them to even consider the possibility of acting responsibly. They will listen to dollars even if they won't listen to reason.

USE YOU ANGER

As you learn more and more about the effects of sugar and the fact that processed food companies have deliberately used their knowledge to addict you to their products - how do you feel about that?

Are you angry?

When you discover how the sugar workers and their children are abused so the sugar companies can make a few extra dollars - do you want to avenge them?

In a futile attempt to grow more and cheaper corn for High Fructose Corn Syrup the agro-industrial giants like Monsanto are poisoning the planet and rendering the human race infertile - does that make you want to take to the streets and protest?

Use your anger to stop the Evil Empire and break your addiction. [4]March Against Monsanto before it's too late.

---

4   http://www.march-against-monsanto.com

Section 4
Corporate Complicity

The average US supermarket sells almost 40,000 products but the vast majority are supplied by just ten companies. P&G, General Mills, Coca Cola, Pepsico, Kellogg's, Mars, Unilever, Kraft, Nestlé, Johnson & Johnson.

The Evil Empire Changes The Game

Now that we know how it is all supposed to work and how it has worked for thousands of years, enter the Evil Empire. Their insatiable desire for profit at any cost changes the game.

In this book we concentrate on the effect that sugar, and particularly fructose, has on our health. But we must also factor in the damage done by pollution, genetic manipulation and stress brought on by Wall Street's greed.

Despite the Empire's attempts to discredit the work of Dr. Lustig and others, more and more reputable scientists are lining up to support his conclusions. The only dissenting voices seem to be those that have something to lose should the truth become well known.

THE IMPACT OF THE "BLISS POINT"

Some of us have heard the term, "the bliss point", but many of us have not. Just what is it and how does it affect our choices?

The food giants actually engineer their processed foods with precisely the right amount of sugar and/or salt and/or fat that will send our senses into absolute bliss. Any nutritional considerations are secondary to a taste that is so compelling that it not only keeps us coming back for more, but may actually make us feel hungrier.

Once again, this smacks of the same tactics used by the tobacco industry to hook consumers by artificially increasing the amount of nicotine. Is this really any different?

The Meeting

The meeting that took place in Minneapolis on April 8, 1999 was unprecedented. The attendees represented a veritable laundry list of the major food companies:

◊ Pillsbury (hosting the meeting)

◊ Nestlé

◊ Kraft

◊ Nabisco

◊ General Mills

◊ Procter & Gamble

◊ Coca Cola

◊ Mars

◊ Cargill

◊ Tate & Lyle

Why had these otherwise fierce competitors, along with two of their major suppliers (Cargill and Tate & Lyle), agreed to this meeting? What was so important that they would feel compelled to discuss anything with the companies they were trying to trounce in the grocery stores?

According to Michael Moss' best selling book, *Salt Sugar Fat: How The Food Giants Hooked Us*, the meeting was organized to address the growing concern over the rising rates of childhood obesity and the impact that the food industry may be having on these statistics.

So, as far back as 1999, the food industry knew there was a growing problem, knew their industry was being scrutinized as a large part of the problem and knew that they should take a look at problem as a group, not just as individual companies.

This meeting was not documented in any way, nothing was recorded, no minutes were taken. What was the outcome of the meeting? Nothing! Just business as usual with the food companies absolving themselves of any guilt for the growing obesity crisis that continues unabated today.

We cannot express the detail, scope, or outcome, of this meeting as eloquently as Michael Moss did in his book and we encourage you to take the time to read it.

Where does packaged food come from - who produces it?

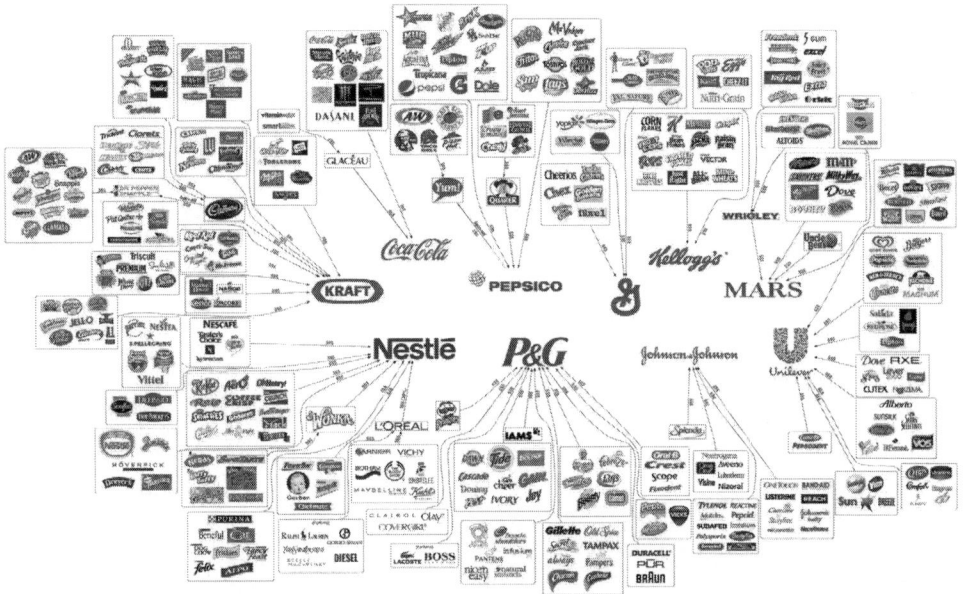

You can find this graphic at many places on the web, here is a link to it on the Huffington Post.

http://www.huffingtonpost.com/2012/04/27/consumer-brands-owned-ten-companies-graphic_n_1458812.html

This image is not up-to-date but it graphically indicates how a small group of people have almost total control over what we are eating.

BUT I EAT ORGANIC

Great! But that doesn't mean we can escape the clutches of the Evil Empire that easily. The industrial giants are buying up organic brands as fast as they can. Brands that built their reputations on providing healthy, nutritious food are being swallowed by multi-nationals who are gradually transforming them into their usual high-profit garbage.

An article from Forbes Magazine on the subject of who owns the organic brands includes a graphic that shows how big food is taking over the organic food market.

http://www.forbes.com/sites/bethhoffman/2013/05/25/

who-owns-organic-brands-and-why-you-should-care/

Here's the link for a larger version of the graphic:

https://www.msu.edu/~howardp/

OrganicMay2013zoom.png

Conventionally Grown vs Organically Grown

Subsidies

Conventional farming (aka agribusiness, aka the Evil Empire) gets all the government subsidies that are going and continually lobbies for more and more.

Most organic farmers are not eligible for any government subsidies.

The Negative Impact Of The Subsidies

Because big agribusiness gets all of the subsidies, particularly on corn (much of which is used for the production of High Fructose Corn Syrup), they can sell their product very, very cheaply. So the processed food industry can also make their food-like products very cheaply.

Organic farmers, even though they are able to produce more yield per acre than the huge conglomerates that use GMO seeds and a dizzying array of chemicals, have to bear the entire cost of their food production without any government help.

This results is a totally insane world in which a McDonald's hamburger can cost only $1.00 but a head of organically grown broccoli can cost $3.00 or more.

It's no wonder that families struggling to survive (once again, thanks to the low wage practices of the Evil Empire) resort to feeding their family at McDonald's, or some other fast food joint, even though they know it's bad for them. They simply can't afford the food that is good for them because those items don't get government subsidies to make them more affordable.

The system is totally backwards when our tax dollars are supporting huge companies that supply us with garbage.

Health Care and The Pharmaceutical Companies

It's no surprise, then, that we are getting sicker and sicker as a result of eating low-nutrition, high-sugar, low-fiber, high calorie processed foods.

Reports show that the rise in [1]type 2 diabetes, heart disease, [2]obesity and more mirror the rise in sugar consumption, not just in the United States, but around the world.

And, the pharmaceutical companies are right on top of developing medications for these chronic diseases. But how can we believe that they have our best interests at heart? What would compel them to try to find a CURE for any of these chronic diseases?

Any cure would seriously impact their bottom line. Don't forget for one minute that their primary purpose is to produce profit for their shareholders. If all the chronic diseases were cured, who would they sell their drugs to?

Documentation Requirements of Conventional Farming vs Organic Farming

Yet another unbelievable, to us anyway, scenario is the documentation requirements for conventional farming in contrast to the requirements for organic farming.

For conventional farming practices it is ASSUMED that the farm will use chemical fertilizers, pesticides and herbicides. It doesn't seem to matter that all of these products are poisonous not only to the plants and insects they are trying to kill, but to other wildlife and, most importantly, to bees. Without bees a lot of our crops would not get pollinated. If they're not pollinated, there are no crops to harvest. A dire situation that we seem to be ignoring.

We also seem to ignore the fact that conventional farming practices spray all kinds of poisons on the food we consume. It is naive to assume that we can simply wash off all these hazardous chemicals.

---

1   http://www.huffingtonpost.com/2013/02/28/sugar-type-2-diabe-tes-rates-robert-lustig_n_2750965.html
2   http://www.theguardian.com/society/2013/mar/20/sugar-deadly-obesity-epidemic

[3]Strict guidelines and documentation are required of organic farmers in order for them to prove that they ARE NOT using the chemicals that the huge agribusiness conglomerates use in alarming quantities, along with other requirements and documentation.

And, in this book, we aren't even addressing GMO seeds which conventional farming can use.

It's simply not a level playing field, making it more cost effective to provide food that this bad for us, cheaply, rather than providing food that has the health benefits that we need.

Although the scope of this book is not to expose the chemicals used in conventional farming, or the GMOs that are grown, it is something that we all should be aware of.

---

3   http://en.wikipedia.org/wiki/Organic_certification

Effects Beyond The USA

As more and more countries around the world adopt a "Western" diet, they, too, are suffering from the effects of all the added sugars in processed foods.

Just like us, they get lured in by the convenience and the taste. And, as we have learned, the taste is carefully engineered to trigger our "bliss point" and keep us, and now the rest of the world, coming back for more.

Incredible as it may seem, there are now more obese people (1.5 billion) than undernourished people (925 million), in the world, according to a [4]Forbes.com article in 2011.

As the rest of the world embraces the "Western lifestyle" they are also realizing the effects of that lifestyle, such as [5]obesity, heart disease, type 2 diabetes and more. And, even though we are now regularly living *longer, our quality of life has suffered as we have to deal with these chronic diseases as we age.

Other countries are obviously not doing themselves any favors by turning to processed and packaged foods. And, for that matter, neither are we.

*By "we are living longer", we mean us, the baby boomers. Those of us lucky enough to have been born before the 1960s. As for our kids, according to the [6]American Heart Association, they have the distinction of being the first generation in history to have a shorter life expectancy than their parents.

---

4   http://www.forbes.com/sites/timworstall/2011/09/22/there-are-now-more-obese-people-than-hungry-people/

5   http://www.cnn.com/2012/12/13/health/global-burden-report/

6   https://www.heart.org/HEARTORG/GettingHealthy/HealthierKids/ChildhoodObesity/Overweight-in-Children_UCM_304054_Article.jsp

Many people don't know that there is a strong connection between Big Tobacco and Big Food - two huge branches of the Evil Empire.

It is sometimes hard to keep track of, and often even harder to find, the connections. Some of the tobacco companies have "spun off" the food companies to try to lessen the connections but many of the executives remain the same.

A few of the more obvious connections that we have been able to uncover are the links between [7]R J Reynolds and Nabisco and [8]Philip Morris (now Altria) and both Kraft and General Foods

HOW THE FOOD INDUSTRY IS EMPLOYING THE SAME TACTICS AS THE TOBACCO INDUSTRY

[9]In an interview with Kelly D. Brownell, the director of the Rudd Center for Food Policy and Obesity at Yale University, he explains to Yale Environment 360 that Big Food is using similar tactics that were employed by Big Tobacco. These tactics included such things as:

◊ employing intense marketing programs aimed at children and young adults

◊ denying that their products are harmful or addictive

◊ denouncing peer-reviewed studies as junk science if there is an suggestion of link between harmful effects and their products

◊ paying scientists for studies showing their products in a favorable light

◊ promising to regulate their own industry or provide healthier options

◊ trying to squash any regulations for labelling, etc. by spending copious amounts of money on lobbying

---

7   http://en.wikipedia.org/wiki/R._J._Reynolds_Tobacco_Company
8   http://abcnews.go.com/Business/story?id=88088
9   http://e360.yale.edu/feature/food_industry_pursues_the_strategy_of_big_tobacco/2136/

A similar article at harvard.edu, [10]*Catch Me If You Can: Big Food Using Big Tobacco's Playbook? Applying the Lessons Learned from Big Tobacco to Attack the Obesity Epidemic*, echoes the sentiments of the Yale article and we encourage you to read both.

PROCESSED FOOD COMPANIES FACING THE SAME LAWYERS THAT BEAT THE TOBACCO COMPANIES

[11]Some of the lawyers that forced tobacco companies to atone, to the cost of several billion dollars, are now actively pursuing suits against Big Food for very much the same reasons.

One such lawyer, Don Barrett, believes regulators have been too soft on the processed food industry and he simply wants these companies to obey already existing laws and tell the truth about what's in their products.

It appears that there is a backlash against a lot of processed foods, particularly those sweetened with High Fructose Corn Syrup, much like we saw against the tobacco industries. An informative article on CNBC.com, [12]*Sugar: The Food Industry's tobacco moment?*, states that although it may not be exactly like the tobacco backlash, there certainly are similarities with calls for companies to be accountable for the effects of their products.

DO WE REALLY WANT TO BE BUYING OUR FOOD FROM TOBACCO COMPANIES?

Many of us don't realize that a lot of the familiar brands we purchase on a regular basis are produced by food companies that are either owned by, or have very close relations with, a tobacco company.

---

10   http://nrs.harvard.edu/urn-3:HUL.InstRepos:8965631

11   http://charlotte.cbslocal.com/2012/10/16/lawyers-who-beat-big-tobacco-now-after-food-industry-companies/

12   http://www.cnbc.com/id/101112144

[13] Adbusters.com has created a page that shows us some of the products that we probably don't know come from just such companies. Some of these products include:

◊ Minute Rice™

◊ Cracker Barrel™ Cheese Products

◊ Jello™

◊ Shake and Bake™

◊ Miracle Whip™

◊ Lunchables™

◊ .... and more!

---

13   https://www.adbusters.org/content/tobacco-food-products

Brainwashing by Advertising and Interest Groups

MARKETING SUGARY FOOD PRODUCTS TO KIDS

In the [14]HBO special, **The Weight of the Nation**, they have made the case that food marketing is connected to unhealthy diets and obesity.

Of particular concern is the marketing of sugar-laden, calorie-dense junk foods to children and young adults. It is estimated that $1.6 billion dollars is allocated, each year, by the food industry specifically, to market to young people.

Advertising to kids becomes even more troubling by the findings that many children have difficulty distinguishing between actual content and advertising. Very young children are not able to tell the difference at all.

According to kidshealth.org, [15]*"Under the age of 8 years, most kids don't understand that commercials are for selling a product. Children 6 years and under are unable to distinguish program content from commercials, especially if their favorite character is promoting the product. Even older kids may need to be reminded of the purpose of advertising."*

FOOD INDUSTRY LOBBYING

Unfortunately, it's a case of whoever has the deepest pockets will prevail in the war over any attempt at regulating the food industry. And, yes, you guessed it, the food industry has the deepest pockets and, apparently, the most resolve as well.

According to a [16]Reuters *Special Report: How Washington went soft on childhood obesity*, Big Food (aka the Evil Empire) is definitely winning the war with many cities, states and even Washington DC, either giving in or

14   https://theweightofthenation.hbo.com/themes/marketing-food-to-children

15   http://kidshealth.org/PageManager.jsp?dn=KidsHealth&lic=1&ps=107&cat_id=&article_set=21720

16   http://www.reuters.com/article/2012/04/27/us-usa-foodlobby-idUSBRE83Q0ED20120427

giving up in the face of overwhelming resistance from the food industry and their lobbyists.

As government agencies have tried to initiate programs and/or regulations to limit the amount of sugar, along with salt and fat, in the food marketed specifically to children, they have been defeated at every turn. During this time frame Big Food has more than doubled their spending in Washington in order to defeat such efforts.

Even Tom Harkin, chairman of the Senate Health committee and a Democrat, says he is upset with the White House for backing down from the fight. Tom Harkin also agrees that the food industry has employed many of the same tactics as Big Tobacco did to fight regulation of the industry. No surprise there because, as we know, there are some close connections between Big Food and Big Tobacco.

The food industry not only uses money, but threats to move the production plants, in order to get the Congress and the Senate to see things their way. Constituents that are afraid of losing their jobs if the food companies pull out will likely not vote their representative back into office. Those in Congress and the Senate are well aware of that fact.

It feels like a battle that just can't be won on a platform of simply what is good for our children and for us, too. Big Food will fight with everything they've got to protect their bottom line.

Once again, the only way we can win is to vote with our dollars. Don't buy their poison and they'll be forced to stop selling it.

The Role of Sugar As A Food Additive

Sugar isn't added to processed foods just to sweeten it, it has several other duties as well.

Here's why sugar is added to processed foods for reasons other than simply sweetening the product:

◊ it aids in browning - also known as the [17]Maillard Reaction

◊ [18]it provides bulk

◊ it adds taste, not just sweetness

◊ it prevents mold from forming

◊ it acts as a preservative

These are some of the reasons that added sugar (in various forms) is found in products that we would not expect to find sugar at all.

Here's a very short list of where added sugars can be lurking:

◊ condiments such as ketchup, some mustards, bbq sauce, [19]Miracle Whip™

◊ salad dressings, even "reduced calorie" dressings

◊ many pasta sauces

◊ sugar alcohols are often added to [20]toothpaste - that's right - toothpaste!

◊ snack chips like [21]Doritos™ and [22]Pringles™ - often in the form of maltodextrin, dextrose or corn syrup solids.

◊ luncheon meats[23]

---

17   http://en.wikipedia.org/wiki/Maillard_reaction
18   http://www.betterhealth.vic.gov.au/bhcv2/bhcarticles.nsf/pages/Sugar
19   http://en.wikipedia.org/wiki/Miracle_Whip#Ingredients
20   http://en.wikipedia.org/wiki/Toothpaste
21   http://en.wikipedia.org/wiki/Doritos#Ingredients
22   http://en.wikipedia.org/wiki/Pringles#Ingredients
23   http://www.today.com/id/16361276/ns/today-today_food/t/

Different Names For Sugar?

[24]Sugar is the generalized name for a class of chemically-related sweet-flavored substances, most of which are used as food. They are carbohydrates, composed of carbon, hydrogen and oxygen.

SUGAR, BY ANY OTHER NAME ...

The word "sugar" is often used as a catch-all phrase for many different forms of sweeteners that are used alone, for food production or as a food additive. In order to make informed choices when reading nutrition labels and ingredient lists, we need to know sugar's other names.

In the ingredient lists of many processed foods we will often see these names listed as separate items. Don't be fooled, they are all still sugar.

Sucrose

(aka Sugar, White Sugar, Table Sugar, Granulated Sugar, Beet Sugar)

Sucrose is the sugar that most of us are familiar with. It is 50% glucose and 50% fructose. It can be derived either from sugar cane or sugar beets.
  ▶ *Fructose Warning: 50% fructose*
  ▶ *GMO Warning: Most sugar beets grown in the United States and Canada are GMO. Check the label when you purchase sugar. If it doesn't say cane sugar then it is most likely made from sugar beets and, as mentioned above, in North America it is most likely from GMO sugar beets. GMO sugar beets are illegal in the rest of the world.*

Fructose

Table sugar (sucrose) is 50% fructose and 50% glucose. The fructose found in whole fruits and vegetables is not particularly harmful because it is being consumed along with fiber, micronutrients, etc.

---

things-you-need-know-about-deli-meats/#.U0f9-seKzsc
24   http://en.wikipedia.org/wiki/Sugar

However, fructose in things like high fructose corn syrup is not accompanied by fiber and/or other nutrients and is metabolized differently, putting a strain on our liver.

▶ *Fructose Warning: Fructose in any form, other than in a whole fruit, is bad for us.*

Glucose

(aka Dextrose or Grape Sugar)

[25]Glucose is metabolized by every cell in our body. It is what our body uses for fuel and does not put a heavy load on our liver like fructose and ethanol do.

THE OTHER NAMES OF SUGAR

Here's a list of names that may be used in the ingredient lists of processed foods, or sold as stand-alone products, and a little information about each of them, including some warnings about fructose levels and the possibility that they may be derived from GMO crops.

Agave Nectar & Agave Syrup

It is hard to nail down the exact percentage of fructose in agave syrup or nectar. Our research found sources that stated the fructose content ranging anywhere from 47% to a whopping 90%! An article in the [26]Huffington Post even claims it is worse than High Fructose Corn Syrup.

▶ *Fructose Warning: High Fructose*

Barley Malt & Barley Malt Syrup

An unrefined sweetener that is very low in Fructose (about 2%) and is sometimes used in brewing and baking.

---

25   http://en.wikipedia.org/wiki/Glucose

26   http://www.huffingtonpost.com/dr-mercola/agave-this-sweetener-is-f_b_537936.html

Brown Rice Syrup

The fructose content of brown rice syrup may be close to 0%.

It's interesting to note that the word "brown" refers to the color of the syrup and not to brown rice. White rice is normally used to make brown rice syrup.

Brown Sugar

Brown sugar is simply regular sugar with molasses added. Therefore, just like regular sugar, it is 50% fructose, 50% glucose. (See Sucrose)
  ▶ *Fructose Warning: 50% fructose*

Cane Sugar

Sugar derived from sugar cane as opposed to sugar beets. (See Sucrose)
  ▶ *Fructose Warning: 50% fructose*

Cane Juice and Cane Juice Crystals

Cane juice is pressed from sugar cane and Cane Juice Crystals are made from evaporated cane juice. They are both essentially the same as white sugar and, therefore, 50% fructose and 50% glucose. (See Sucrose)
  ▶ *Fructose Warning: 50% fructose*

[27]Carob Syrup

It appears that carob syrup is about the same as sucrose - 50% fructose, 50% glucose.
  ▶ *Fructose Warning: 50% fructose*

Confectioner's Sugar

Often referred to as powdered sugar or icing sugar, it is also Sucrose. (see Sucrose).
  ▶ *Fructose Warning: 50% fructose*

---

27   http://www.livestrong.com/article/253042-which-sugars-does-carob-contain/

Corn Syrup

Regular corn syrup should not be confused with High Fructose Corn Syrup (HFCS). They are NOT the same. Real corn syrup is made from corn starch and has no fructose. Regular corn syrup may also be called Glucose Syrup.

Although regular corn syrup is glucose, it still has almost the same calories per teaspoon as sugar (sugar = 15 calories/teaspoon, corn syrup = 20 calories/teaspoon, "lite" corn syrup = 13 calories/teaspoon), but it is not very sweet.

▶ *GMO Warning: May be produced using GMO corn.*

High Fructose Corn Syrup

High fructose corn syrup may be called by other names in different countries, such as glucose/fructose (Canada), Isoglucose, Glucose-Fructose syrup and high-fructose maize syrup (Europe).

▶ *Fructose Warning: 55% Fructose*
▶ *GMO Warning: May be produced from GMO corn*

Corn Sweetener

Don't be fooled by the term corn sweetener, it is just another name for High Fructose Corn Syrup.

▶ *Fructose Warning: 55% Fructose*
▶ *GMO Warning: May be produced from GMO corn*

Corn Syrup Solids

Corn syrup solids are derived from regular corn syrup, not high fructose corn syrup. If high fructose corn syrup is used, it must be labeled as such. Corn syrup solids in an ingredient list is made from regular corn syrup and is, therefore, mostly dextrose (glucose).

▶ *GMO Warning: May be produced from GMO corn.*

Crystallized Fructose

According to Wikipedia, [28]crystalline fructose is at least 98% pure fructose and is derived from corn. It is used in beverages and yogurts and is used in place of HFCS (High Fructose Corn Syrup) or table sugar (sucrose).

▶ *Fructose Warning: 98% fructose*

▶ *GMO Warning: may be produced from GMO corn*

Date Sugar

Our research did not produce much information on date sugar. [29]Wikipedia has a tiny article that gives little information. It appears that it is made from pulverized dried dates, and nothing else, and is frequently available in health food stores. To date we have been unable to find a reliable source to show the breakdown of the glucose/fructose content. However, as dates are a fruit, there will, of course, be fructose in date sugar.

Evaporated Cane Juice

Is essentially the same as regular white sugar. (see Sucrose)

▶ *Fructose Warning: 50% fructose*

Fruit Juice

Fruit juice is often included on processed food ingredients labels but is not necessarily called a "sugar". Added fruit juice is often devoid of its accompanying fiber, making the sugar impact much larger. Naturally, fruit juice will have fructose (fruit sugar). The amount of fructose will vary by the type of fruit.

▶ *Fructose Warning: Unknown percentage of fructose.*

Fruit Juice Concentrate

This is just what it sounds like - fruit juice concentrated. In order to make the juice in the first place, generally all the fiber is removed in the

---

28   http://en.wikipedia.org/wiki/Crystalline_fructose
29   http://en.wikipedia.org/wiki/Date_sugar

process. Then, to make concentrate, most of the water is removed, not only concentrating the juice, but the sugars as well.

▶ *Fructose Warning: Unknown percentage of fructose.*

Glucose Solids

Glucose solids are powdered glucose. (See Glucose)

Golden Sugar

Golden sugar is simply white sugar with some molasses or refining syrup added. (See Sucrose)

Golden Syrup or Refiner's Syrup

This is a thick, amber-colored form of inverted sugar syrup. (See Sucrose)

Grape Juice Concentrate

Grape juice concentrate is sometimes used as a food additive and is exactly what it sounds like - concentrated grape juice.

▶ *Fructose Warning: Unknown percentage of fructose.*

Honey

Honey contains both glucose and sucrose, along with several other beneficial compounds, including anti-oxidants.

▶ *Warning: When purchasing honey, be sure to get real honey. There are many commercial honeys, particularly those from China, where some of the honey has been replaced by high fructose corn syrup or other sweeteners.*

▶ *Fructose Warning: Some of the commercially produced honey may contain High Fructose Corn Syrup.*

▶ *GMO Warning: Any High Fructose Corn Syrup present in honey may be produced using GMO corn.*

Invert Sugar

Invert sugar, or invert sugar syrup, is a mixture of glucose and fructose that is derived from sucrose and is frequently used for baked goods. (see Sucrose)

▶ *Fructose Warning: 50% fructose*

▶ *GMO warning: if the sugar used is derived from sugar beets grown in North America, chances are that the sugar beets are GMO.*

Lactose

Lactose is also known as milk sugar. It is comprised of galactose and glucose. Providing your body produces the enzyme lactase the galactose is converted to glucose.

Maltodextrin or Malt or Maltose

This form of sugar is frequently found in processed foods. Our body will convert it to glucose.

Maple Syrup

Maple syrup can be made from several species of maple trees but is usually made from the sap of sugar maple, red maple or black maple trees, although it can also be made from other maple species. Maple syrup may be one of the least processed and healthier sweeteners we can use.

Molasses or Treacle

Molasses (American & Canadian) or treacle (British) is a viscous by-product of the refining of sugarcane, grapes, or sugar beets into sugar.

▶ *Fructose Warning: 50% fructose*

▶ *GMO Warning: may be made with GMO beets*

Raw Sugar

According to food.com, [30]raw sugar is the residue left after sugarcane has been processed to remove the molasses and refine the sugar crystals. Genuinely raw sugar contains molds and fibers which are considered nutrients, however, according to the [31]Canadian Sugar Institute, raw sugar is not sold to consumers because it doesn't meet Canadian Standards for health and hygiene. In North America, sugar claiming to be "raw" has been processed and is, therefore, sucrose. (see Sucrose).

Sorghum Syrup

Sweet sorghum syrup is sometimes confused with molasses but it is not the same thing. Molasses is a by-product of sugar production, whereas sorghum syrup is made from the juice of the sorghum cane and is not a by-product. Much like maple syrup, sorghum juice is boiled down to produce the syrup. It takes about ten gallons of sorghum juice to make about one gallon of sorghum syrup. This syrup contains both glucose and fructose, much like sucrose but does not have any dietary fiber. (See Sucrose)

▶ **Fructose Warning: 36% fructose**

Sucanat

Sucanat is actually a brand name for a type of whole cane sugar. In essence it is dried sugar cane juice that has retained its molasses content. (See Sucrose)

GOOD REFERENCE WEBSITE

During our research, we found the website by the Canadian Sugar Institute to be a good resource for comparing the different types and names of sugar. We encourage you to visit -

http://www.sugar.ca/english/consumers/typessugar.cfm

---

30   http://www.food.com/library/raw-sugar-484
31   http://www.sugar.ca/Nutrition-Information-Service/Consumers/About-Sugar/Types-of-Sugar.aspx

OUR RESEARCH

Finding all of the different names for sugar has been challenging to say the least. This is the most comprehensive list and explanations we were able to put together. There still may be more names that the food industry uses to hide all the added sugars used in processed foods.

SOME RULES TO CONSIDER

Several good rules of thumb when purchasing foods are:

◊ If you don't recognize the ingredient, or can't pronounce it, you probably don't want it in your food.

◊ If it doesn't go bad, it's probably bad for you (Twinkies come to mind). If it can go bad, it's probably good for you (like fresh fruits and vegetables).

◊ If it has a television commercial, or any other types of mass media advertising, odds are you don't want it.

◊ And, it should go without saying, most fast food establishments should be avoided.

Beware Of Misleading Food Labels

Packaged food companies are fully aware of the growing movements towards healthier diets and away from the food-like products they have been pushing for the past quarter century. Of course this does not mean they plan to change their ways, only that they will change their marketing message.

REDUCED FAT OR FAT FREE

In order to reduce, or eliminate, fat in processed foods, most companies add in more sugar and often more salt and/or artificial or natural flavors to compensate.

It is often assumed, as well, that these products are low in calories. Don't be fooled - they're not. Take the time to read the labels. Better yet, just put them back on the shelf.

LITE OR LIGHT

As far as we can tell from the [32]FDA website, the most common allowed use of "lite" or "light" means that the product has at least 50% less fat than the comparable "regular" product. Or it can have at least one-third few calories than the "regular" product.

HEALTHY

The [33]FDA requirements for being able to label a product as "healthy" are quite lengthy and, at times, a little confusing. Our best suggestion here would be to be skeptical about any such claims on processed foods. We should decide for ourselves what is and isn't healthy and not let the Evil Empire tell us what that is.

---

32   http://www.accessdata.fda.gov/scripts/cdrh/cfdocs/cfcfr/CFRSearch.cfm?fr=101.56
33   http://www.accessdata.fda.gov/scripts/cdrh/cfdocs/cfcfr/CFRSearch.cfm?fr=101.65

SECTION 5 LIVING WITH SUGAR

AN INTRODUCTION TO A SUGAR FREE DIET?

Humans crave sweet, it's part of who we are and we can't ignore it. The theory is that our ancestors determined that if a food was sweet it was not poisonous so, therefore, it was good to eat. Big Food exploits this natural craving by adding just the right amount of cheap sugar to make their products irresistible.

Sugar in Our Culture

In a little over 200 years, sugar has insinuated itself not only into our diets but also our culture.

Our Holidays, Events and Celebrations

◊ What's Halloween without candies?

◊ What's Valentine's Day without chocolates?

◊ What's a birthday without a cake with lots of sugary icing?

◊ What's Christmas without candies and plum pudding?

◊ What's a trip to the fair without indulging in some candy floss or caramel corn?

Firmly Planted In Our Lexicon

◊ Who hasn't said, I'm not going to sugar coat this for you?

◊ Many parents, us included, have combined crushed medicine with sugar or a sugary jam because we believed in the saying a spoonful of sugar helps the medicine go down, immortalized in the Disney film, Mary Poppins.

◊ Terms of endearment include: sugar, sweet as sugar, sugar pie, cupcake. We're sure you can come up with many more.

In Our Cooking and Baking

◊ In many kitchens, sugar is the first thing we reach for if we're planning to make pies, jams, preserves, cakes, cookies and even bread.

◊ Maybe it's time to turn the clock back and eradicate not only the sugar but the use of such terms in everyday language. Yes, perhaps our language will be less rich, but we will have eliminated a poison.

Just How Much Sugar Is In Our Food

When we read the "Nutrition" labels on packaged foods we find the sugar content of a product serving expressed in grams. The first thing to note is that the listed "serving size" is usually totally unrealistic. Who eats just one cookie?

It's also unlikely that we can visualize what a gram of sugar looks like, unless we're a lab technician. One teaspoon of sugar is roughly equal to 4 grams. That Big Drink at the convenience store has 128 grams of sugar or 32 teaspoons, around 512 calories. If our daily caloric intake should be less than 2000, we just drank more than a quarter of our daily calorie allowance.

SHOW ME THE SUGAR

When you read the paragraph above you probably said something like, "Wow, that's a lot of sugar." But you may still not be sure what that much sugar looks like. Fortunately the folks at http://www.sugarstacks.com have solved that problem for us by photographing various food and drink items beside a pile of the cubes of sugar they contain.

When we look at the photos on their site we start to understand how impossible it is to avoid sugar if we eat a traditional North American diet.

CUTTING OUT THE SUGAR

The goal is not to eliminate sugar from your diet because "sugar" is the fuel that powers your muscles. Starch in the form of a potato or slice of bread is immediately turned into glucose by your body and burned by your mitochondria. The goal is to eliminate the ADDED sugar found in processed food.

The Paleo Diet

The Paleo diet has been getting a lot of attention lately as a way to eat that is in line with the way we evolved. We certainly applaud the theory but in practice the way people choose to implement it has little to do with the diet of our Paleolithic ancestors.

Unless we believe The Flintstones was a documentary, most of us can be pretty certain early man didn't drive to the supermarket, eat bacon for breakfast, sausages for lunch and corn fed steak for supper.

We are not suggesting that grass fed meat in moderation is bad for us but three meals a day of the chemical laden muck the meat industry is foisting onto an unsuspecting public today has little to do with meat of even fifty years ago.

Our meat animals are fed subsidized GMO corn because it's cheap. Since they are not designed to eat corn they get sick so we give them antibiotics which have the added benefit of making them fatten up quicker.

In fact, we give our meat animals so many antibiotics that the [1]Union of Concerned scientists estimated 70% of all antibiotics in the U.S. (24.6 million pounds annually) are fed to livestock and not taken by people.

At least we're not taking them directly but, of course, if we eat the meat we also get the second hand antibiotics.

But if we truly follow a Paleolithic diet AND WAY OF LIFE of our ancestors then we would be following the lifestyle we are best adapted to. The downside, of course, is that life was pretty brutal back then and we were unlikely to live much beyond our 20s.

So what can we do today that allows us to live a long and healthy life and enjoy the rich taste experiences available to modern humans?

---

1   http://www.ucsusa.org/assets/documents/food_and_agriculture/ hog_front.pdf

Vegetarians And Sugar

Deciding to become a vegetarian is a good first step but we should not assume that a vegetarian diet is intrinsically healthy. There are many foods that are vegetarian and are most definitely not good to eat, sugar being one of them.

A vegetarian can drink gallons of sugar laden soft drinks and still be vegetarian. Cakes, cookies and candy bars can all be vegetarian, even ice cream is vegetarian although not vegan because it is made with milk.

There are no dietary restrictions for any natural or artificial sweeteners because none of them are animal based.

Vegetarians don't have to worry about staying away from sugar cured ham and bacon or all the other cured meats that contain sugar but they do need to read the labels on any processed food they buy.

Sugar coated cereals are vegetarian as is ketchup and canned fruit but they are all high in sugar.

Unfortunately, following a vegetarian or vegan diet will not protect us from consuming toxic quantities of sugar. Vegetarians must be just as vigilant as everyone else if they are to avoid the consequences of dietary sugar.

A Reduced Sugar Diet

We will start by defining what we mean by diet. In the context of this section we mean diet as a lifestyle not as a means to lose weight. There is a very good chance that you will lose weight when you follow our suggestions but the goal is to eat healthier and not gain unwanted belly fat as the years go by.

If your goal is to lose weight this is a good place to start but you will need to monitor your intake more closely, avoid snacks and be sure to get the proper exercise.

MAJOR CHANGES

If you are serious about following a healthy lifestyle it's not that difficult but there are a couple of major changes that most people will need to make.

EATING

1. Cut out all soft drinks and fruit juices.
2. Eliminate all "Fast Food".
3. Eat fresh prepared food not convenient imitation food.
4. Reduce or eliminate the amount of meat you eat.
5. Increase the amount of fibre in your diet.
6. Drink no more than 1 or 2 glasses of red wine a day.
7. Snack on fresh fruit and nuts instead of cookies and candy.

EXERCISE

We have already established that you won't lose weight by exercising but regular exercise is critical to a healthy lifestyle. Not only is exercise important but the time of day you exercise can make a tremendous difference to your results.

Counting Calories

If you have not already read our discussion about calories in the medical section we urge you to read that first before continuing.

We have established that not all calories are the same. Fructose calories and alcohol calories do you more harm than carbohydrate calories because of the way they are metabolized. But even "good" calories still count in our body's energy balance sheet.

Food calories are calculated using a device called a bomb calorimeter which actually burns the food and a measurement is taken of the rise in temperature of the water in a chamber that surrounds the food. The food is reduced to ash, which of course our bodies do not do and a food high in fiber will obviously give a false reading because our bodies do not consume fiber.

All problems aside the calorie, or European kilojoules, are the only universal measurements we have of the potential effects of different foods.

So our advice is to use the information given by the calorie count but to apply some additional common sense before putting the food in our mouths.

We now know which foods are bad for us and, most importantly, why. The smart thing to do is avoid the bad foods regardless of the number of calories they contain.

For example 100 grams of almonds contains 576 calories and a chocolate donut has around 452 calories. We can easily eat a donut but we would find it difficult to eat 100 grams of almonds. Even if we could eat more than a cupful of almonds in one go it would still be healthier than eating the chocolate donut.

So, the bottom line here is to absolutely count calories so we can monitor our intake but only eat foods that will metabolize to glucose. Avoid the fructose and alcohol.

Soft Drinks And Fruit Juices

If we do nothing else we must eliminate soft drinks, fruit juices and other sweetened beverages from our diet. This is absolutely the most critical step we can take towards a more healthy lifestyle. It may be very difficult because sugar is addictive but the results will be well worth the effort.

There is nothing wrong with municipal water right out of the faucet. At least in most cases. If you live in an area that still fluoridates the water supply or the petroleum division of the Evil Empire is fracking close by and contaminating your water with natural gas, you may have to buy bottled water. You could also get a home filtering system that ranges from a portable Brita jug to an under counter system that requires a plumber to link it into your water supply

A quick Google search for "3rd world water treatment" will find all kinds of innovative solutions for cheap and easy solutions for obtaining potable water from dubious sources.

You can flavor the water with an assortment of fruits, berries, leaves and roots to make vitamin waters and teas.

A popular [2]myth is that, up until modern times, people drank beer rather than water because the brewing process cleaned up the water. There is no truth to this belief and although a cold beer on a hot summer day is a wonderful thing the sugar hit is something we need to be cognizant of.

OK you're right, there's no sugar listed on the beer label but beer is carbs and alcohol and we know from the Medical section what happens when we take in carbs and alcohol. The carbs turn into glucose and the alcohol gets metabolized in our brain and liver. But that is still about a third of the hit from a soft drink, so enjoy - but just one.

---

2   http://leslefts.blogspot.ca/2013/11/the-great-medieval-water-myth.html

No Fast Food

We're talking about burgers, fries, donuts, ice cream and soft drinks, etc. We know this stuff is bad for us so stop eating it. Even in the fast food brand restaurants it is possible to make reasonably healthy choices.

Most of the chains have some sort of salad selection - but choose a vinaigrette dressing rather than one of the creamy ones. Wendy's offers baked potatoes, which is a good choice. Sure the starch will be converted to glucose almost immediately but if we combine it with a salad the roughage will help to slow down the absorption. Glucose isn't the enemy, fructose is.

We can use the Internet to discover the ingredients and nutritional information for every fast food menu in the country. Just type "<CHAIN NAME> nutrition" into a browser search box and find out where the sugar is. We can do the same thing for casual dining chains as well.

You bought a book about sugar so there is a pretty good chance you're overweight. There's also a good chance you eat a lot of crap and drink soft drinks or juice. It's not your fault, you're bombarded daily with millions of dollars worth of advertising to buy these products. The manufacturers of these food-like products know they're bad for us but they don't care, So long as they continue to make obscene profits they will continue to produce the crap. We need to stop supporting the Evil Empire with our dollars and our lives.

Convenience Food

Just what do we mean by "convenience" food? It means different things to different people. But, what we're referring to is stuff that is meant to make meal preparation a little easier. Things like frozen dinners, frozen pizzas, spaghetti sauce, most breads and anything we might pick up for dessert.

And, if you have squeezable cheese, ready cooked spaghetti or instant anything in your cupboards you need to seriously re-evaluate your dietary choices.

Even those of us who do most of their cooking from scratch sometimes get a little help from things like tetra pack vegetable broth. Imagine our surprise when we realized that there is sugar - yes, sugar - in something as simple as vegetable broth, along with a whole bunch of other ingredients that we neither want nor need. Vegetable broth is one of those things that may take a little time to prepare, but you can make lots of it and then freeze it - even in ice cube trays for that time that you only need a little.

If your family sits down to meals together and eats meals prepared from fresh locally grown organic fruits and vegetables, we applaud you. Unfortunately, the vast majority of North American families do none of these things and it shows.

It's a sad fact that most households grab something to eat on the run. For many families the only time they eat together is holidays like Thanksgiving and Christmas.

Convenience foods are making us sick and fat. And being sick and fat isn't all that convenient!

Those warning labels that are now required on cigarette packages should also be required on most of the 40,000 items in the average supermarket. Sugar, salt, fat and GMOs are the major contributor to our growing obesity and chronic disease epidemic.

According to the Centers for Disease Control and Prevention in 2007, national health care expenditures in the United States totaled $2.2 trillion or 16% of its gross domestic product, a 14% increase from 2000. This represents an average of more than $7,400 per person.

By 2020 these figures are expected to more than double to $4.6 trillion.

The amount of money is staggering but remember this represents a nation of very sick people suffering miserable lives caused in large part by what they eat.

We are doing it to ourselves and we need to STOP IT.

We will all benefit from learning to cook, slowing down and taking time for proper meals with our families. Don't eat food that comes in packages.

By the way, we can easily make our own convenience food that doesn't have all the junk in it. Spend a day cooking and packaging up entrées for the freezer. Just add some fresh veggies and potato or pasta and a real meal is ready in twenty minutes, or less. And when we make our own convenience food, we retain all the vitamins, nutrients and fiber, just like nature intended.

Before you toss the next package or can into your shopping cart take a minute to read the label. Now ask yourself if the "convenience" is worth shortening your life or your children's life.

Modern Meat

Old McDonald sold his farm to a huge agribusiness corporation. In the interest of making the maximum profit the new owners crammed all the animals in the smallest space possible.

Corn is really cheap because the farm corporations have bribed the politicians to create huge subsidies that keep the price of corn way below what it actually costs to grow. Even though the animals aren't genetically designed to eat corn it's the cheapest way to feed them and they do fatten up quickly.

They need to fatten up quickly so they can be slaughtered before they die from eating all the corn. Just to be sure, they also get injected with antibiotics which, along with keeping them alive, also helps to put on more weight.

We will have much more to say on this subject in a future Terra Novian report but our advice is to avoid as much meat as you can. We're not radical vegetarians although since animal cruelty laws don't apply to food animals we get very upset when we see the kind of abuse these poor creatures must suffer.

When Old McDonald was running things the animals had a reasonable life, out in the sun, stress free, fresh natural food and a quick death. Now they spend their short lives in daily terror, in the dark and standing in feces.

If you really can't give up your meat, you owe it to yourself and the animals to buy meat that is produced the old fashioned way. It tastes better and you don't get all the chemicals that the large meat producers use.

Old McDonald has changed his name to [3]Polyface. A great example of natural, sustainable farming.

http://www.polyfacefarms.com

---

3   http://www.polyfacefarms.com

Dietary Fiber

We have already written quite a bit about fiber and how important it is in maintaining good health. We wrote that our Paleolithic ancestors ate 100 grams of fiber every day. You should take particular note of this if you are on the Paleo diet because all that meat will really clog up your system.

The human gut is much longer than a carnivore gut and if the meat doesn't pass through quickly it will putrefy and contribute to colon cancer.

So just how much is 100 grams of fiber? It's a lot and we don't actually have to eat that much - the recommended daily dose is only 25 grams but more won't hurt us. [4]Mount Sinai Hospital has produced an excellent section on their website that discusses the importance of fiber in our diet.

They also have a [5]chart that lists the fiber content of various foods.

Take the time to compare your current diet with the items on the chart and there is a good chance you will come up several grams of fiber short.

This is also where the recommendation of 6-8 glasses of water a day comes from. We need the fluid, (coffee, tea, flavoured water) to mix with the fiber and keep it soft as it makes its way through our colon.

The only problem we have with the chart is that it lists a lot of things we shouldn't be eating. Just think of this list as a complete resource and not as a list of recommended items.

---

4   https://www.wehealny.org/healthinfo/dietaryfiber/index.html
5   https://www.wehealny.org/healthinfo/dietaryfiber/fiberContentChart.html

Alcohol Consumption

Alcohol, like sugar, is toxic depending on the dose. Our bodies can handle small quantities but become overwhelmed if the dose is too large.

If you find the idea of your morning coffee without a teaspoon of sugar unthinkable, then you should have it. A teaspoonful is not going to make a difference, (consult your doctor if you are diabetic) and life is too short to stress about it. But if you allow a lot of little indulgences then you will pay the price.

The same goes for alcohol. We have already said that studies show a glass of red wine a day is good for us but the alcohol will still turn to fat.

The same goes for beer and spirits. If you are not trying to lose weight and your system is efficiently burning the calories you consume, then a beer or shot won't do any harm.

We found a chart online that compares alcohol and calorie content for a very impressive number of alcoholic beverages.

https://www.wehealny.org/healthinfo/dietaryfiber/ fiberContentChart.html

Just remember that alcohol does not get metabolized directly by our mitochondria - it turns to fat.

Snack on Fresh Fruit And Nuts

When did snacking become something we did?

By definition it would have to be sometime after we established regular meal times. One thing we can be sure of is that the snack food was made from fresh, wholesome, nutritions ingredients. The sort of things we consider "snack" food didn't start to appear until late in the Victorian era as this article in the Wall Street Journal indicates.

http://online.wsj.com/news/articles/SB1000142412788
732400930457904132266798165O

Today snacking should be looked on as another triumph of the Evil Empire's marketing machine. Sell as much cheap crap as possible for the maximum profit regardless of the damage done to the health of the population.

According to a sample report from [6]First Research worldwide snack food sales generate 300 billion in revenue. This does nor include cookies and candies that are not considered a snack food.

There are two competing theories about snacking. One side says by eating between meals you are less likely to overeat at mealtime but we are unaware of any actual data that supports this position. The truth is that what began as a once in awhile treat has become a daily indulgence.

The scientific side of the snack debate clearly shows that in order to reset our insulin and leptin levels we must cut out snacks and eat nothing for at least four hours before bedtime.

Water or tea is OK providing we don't add milk or sweetener as that would be considered by our body to be food which would cause our pancreas to release insulin.

If you are not trying to lose weight and must eat something between meals then at least make it something like nuts or a piece of fruit. But our best option is to drink some water or brush your teeth - it helps, really.

---

6   https://www.firstresearch.com/industryanalysis/First_Research_
Industry_Profile_Sample.pdf

Exercise Timing

In the exercise section we talked about how important regular exercise is to build glucose-burning mitochondria and turning white fat into brown fat.

We also pointed out that exercise as a direct way to lose weight doesn't work because of our body's efficient use of energy. We need to expand on this a little and explain how we can maximize our exercise efforts.

We discovered in the medical section how our bodies use hormones to communicate and regulate each process. In regards to eating, insulin and leptin are the primary hormones that need to be working properly but for a growing number of the population our bodies are "resistant" to their influence.

The problem is that our digestive system never gets any time off. We eat too much of the wrong foods so our systems are always flooded with insulin. We need to allow our body to finish with one meal before we give it another one to work on. Our Paleolithic ancestors carried their lunch boxes on a hunt as abdominal fat.

Our muscles and liver store glucose as glycogen for immediate use as needed. [7]We have around 2000 kcal available in total but this is spread among different muscles and they are not set up to share. In other words, we have enough stored glycogen energy to run for about a day providing we are not doing any exercise.

This means that our bodies won't dip into their stores of visceral fat until we use up, and don't replenish, our glucose/glycogen levels.

If you do the math it looks like going for a brisk walk before breakfast could be the most productive exercise you can do.

Don't eat anything for at least four hours before you go to sleep. Get a good eight hours of sleep and go for a brisk one hour walk before breakfast.

The next controversy is what to have for breakfast.

---

7   http://www.extension.iastate.edu/humansciences/content/carbo-hydrate

How Do I Break My Fast?

Millions of dollars worth of advertising says you should eat some sort of grain and sugar combination. Often with chocolate, marshmallows, raisins or fake fruit as an added bonus.

DO YOU CARE WHAT YOUR KIDS EAT?

If you do check out the website at:

http://www.cerealfacts.org

You also might like to read the full report they make available at:

http://www.cerealfacts.org/media/Cereal_FACTS_ Report_2012_7.12.pdf

Still not convinced? Here's a British report that list US cereals along with some UK only brands:

http://www.childrensfoodcampaign.net/Which%20 Cereals%20Report%20Feb%202012.pdf

There is absolutely nothing in any of these products to recommend them. You can easily provide your family with a nourishing breakfast that is cheaper, just as convenient and dramatically better for them. Just stop buying this junk!

MAYBE WE SHOULD JUST SKIP BREAKFAST

Research shows that you will probably eat more during the day if you skip breakfast. Certainly never send a kid to school without a good breakfast as the ghrelin grumble signals are hard to ignore. It's hard to learn when you're hungry.

SO WHAT SHOULD WE EAT?

OK, so it's clear that commercial cereals are a really bad idea. How about making your own? We've included our recipe for Homemade, Sugar-Free, Granola in the next section.

But our best choice is a breakfast high in protein because protein does not stimulate insulin production like carbs do and the longer digestion time helps to keep us satiated longer.

GOOD BREAKFAST CHOICES

Homemade, Sugar-Free Granola

Let's start with our Homemade, Sugar-Free Granola. The basic recipe has 10 grams of protein and 8 grams of fiber. Add ½ cup of milk (4 grams) and a 3 oz dollop of greek yogurt (8-10 grams) for a total 24 grams of protein to start your day.

Breakfast Burrito

The combination of a corn tortilla wrapped around two scrambled eggs a ¼ cup of black beans plus a ¼ cup of diced sautéed onions packs a 25 gram protein punch.

Simple Toast

Invest in a bread machine and make your own whole grain breads for half the price of store bought and without all the extra ingredients. (commercial bakers use plaster of Paris as a dough conditioner).

Skip the butter and spread your fresh whole grain toast with 2 tbsp of peanut butter for 10 grams of protein. Get real peanut butter from a bulk food store not the commercial brands that replace the peanut oil with GMO canola oil besides adding other chemicals and, of course, sugar.

Omelets & Frittatas

Combine eggs with cheese, spinach, broccoli, asparagus, salmon and dozens of other assorted healthy ingredients. It's quick, inexpensive and the best way to start the day.

Sugar Alternatives

The message we hope we have conveyed in this book is that sugar is toxic. The larger the dose we get the more damage it does. Our body can deal with small doses of glucose but fructose, other than what is contained in fresh fruit, is something we should avoid.

So what do we do about our "sweet tooth"

As we remove sugar from our diet, our taste buds will more easily be able to recognise 'sweetness'. We will find our sweet tooth is satisfied with a much lower level of sweetness.

Artificial sweeteners are dangerous and seem to have a chemical rather than sweet taste.

Fortunately, there are many natural products that can be substituted for sugar to provide sweetness to our recipes. It's true that the natural products get their sweetness from the same glucose and fructose as sugar so they still need to be used in moderation. The natural products also provide other nutritional benefits not found in processed sugar.

Not A Free Pass

We've said it earlier in this book but it bears repeating - sugar-free does NOT mean calorie-free.

Although the following sweetener alternatives are not sugar, they do have calories and we need to take that into account when using them.

Honey

Honey - real honey - is a natural product that not only supplies sweetness but nutrients and healing properties as well. Unfortunately, we're not being good stewards of our honey bee colonies.

The total disregard for future generations is aptly demonstrated by the Evil Empire's treatment of bees. [8]The quote below, erroneously attributed to Albert Einstein, sums up the problem:

8   http://quoteinvestigator.com/2013/08/27/einstein-bees/

"If the bee disappeared off the surface of the globe then man would only have four years of life left. No more bees, no more pollination, no more plants, no more animals, no more man."

SPECTACULARLY STUPID AND SHORTSIGHTED

The hard working honey bee has been toiling for man for thousands of years. For the most part it has been of a mostly one sided benefit but dedicated beekeepers looked after their hives because their livelihoods depended on it.

The beekeepers still care about their hives for much the same reasons but environmental changes are far beyond the control of the beekeeper and the bees are paying the price.

One practice that is in the control of the beekeeper is their greed to steal the maximum amount of honey from the bees that they possibly can. The bees collect and store honey as food. It is their only motivation. The modern commercial beekeeper often steals all of the honey their bees produce. Then they feed the bees High Fructose Corn Syrup. We know that stuff is bad for us so we can only assume that it is equally bad for the bees.

Some forward-thinking beekeepers leave enough honey behind for the bees to eat. This practice ensures that the bees get proper nutrition by eating what nature intended them to eat and what they have, for millennia, produced for themselves.

Chemically HFCS and Honey are quite similar but it has been found that at temperatures above 45 °C HFCS rapidly becomes toxic. Also HFCS does not contain several ingredients that induce detoxification genes and allow the bees to deal with pesticides and other pathogens they now face.

Calories: 1 teaspoon = 21 Calories

Maple Syrup

Indigenous North American peoples were the first to harvest the sap from Maple trees. The most common species of Maple trees for the best sap production are the Sugar Maple, the Black Maple and the Red Maple. It is possible to tap other species of Maples but the taste will vary.

European settlers followed the example of native Americans and began tapping Maple trees as well.

The highest production of Maple syrup comes for the province of Quebec in Canada, accounting for 75% of all Maple syrup produced worldwide. The second largest producer, at only 5.5%, is the state of Vermont.

According to the [9]Pure Canadian Maple Syrup website, Maple syrup has some amazing benefits including over 54 antioxidants, so these are not just "empty" calories as the calories from sugar are.

Calories: 1 teaspoon = 17 Calories

Corn Syrup

Regular corn syrup is not to be confused with High Fructose Corn Syrup - they are not the same thing. Regular corn syrup is 100% glucose - that's right, the fuel our body uses and needs.

Most of us, if we're used to using sugar or HFCS sweetened foods, will find that regular corn syrup is not very sweet. However, if we make the effort to eliminate those bad sweeteners from our diet, that perception may change.

One caveat, though, is that most corn syrup available today is made from GMO corn and should probably be avoided.

Visit the website for the [10]Non-GMO project for products that do not include GMOs.

Calories: 1 teaspoon = 19 Calories

Dates

Dates have been part of the Middle Eastern diet for thousands of years and are the fruit of the date palm tree.

It's [11]nutritional value is quite impressive, including protein, fiber, calcium, iron and more.

---

9   http://www.purecanadamaple.com/benefits-of-maple-syrup
10   http://www.nongmoproject.org/
11   http://ndb.nal.usda.gov/ndb/foods/show/2277

To be used as a sweetener, dates can simply be chopped up and added to a recipe, as we do in granola. We can also cook chopped dates with a little bit of water and a squeeze of lemon, until it becomes a paste, and then is easily added to recipes requiring a smoother or more liquid type of sweetener.

Calories: 1 date = 23 Calories

Figs

The common fig, the fruit of the Ficus carica, contain [12]flavonoids, natural sugars and vitamins, as well as calcium, iron and more.

Figs can be used either fresh or dried. The dried figs will, of course, have their natural sugars more concentrated.

We can use them as sweeteners using that same method we would for dates. Or, they can, of course, be eaten alone.

Calories: 1 fig = 47 Calories

Prunes

Prunes, also referred to as dried plums, can also be used a sweetener.

Unfortunately, prunes have come to have a somewhat negative connotation as only being useful for the elderly to aid with chronic constipation. That is perhaps why we now seem them referred to as dried plums more frequently than prunes.

Whatever we choose to call them, they are not only lovely and sweet, but they are also good for us, containing [13]fiber, vitamins, iron and more.

Eat them as they are, or prepare them as you would dates or figs.

Calories: 1 prune = 23 Calories

---

12   http://ndb.nal.usda.gov/ndb/foods/show/2284
13   http://ndb.nal.usda.gov/ndb/foods/show/2439

Dried Fruit

There are many other dried fruits that can be used as sweeteners, too many to list here. Sweetness levels and taste will, of course, vary by the fruit chosen.

Experiment with your favorites but make sure to watch the calorie counts, too.

Nuts

We have found that the sweetest nut is the pecan and it can certainly help add sweetness to our recipes.

Be sure to use dry-roasted pecans, as the roasting helps to bring out their flavor and sweetness. Then add them either chopped or ground.

Pecans provide many benefits to our health and diet such as [14]fiber, protein, vitamins, calcium, iron and more.

20 grams of pecans = approximately 1/4 cup = 138 Calories

Explore the use of other nuts, too, just be sure to check their calories.

---

14   http://ndb.nal.usda.gov/ndb/foods/show/3724

Section 6 Cooking Without Sugar

This section is included to inspire a new way of looking at cooking without the use of sugar. It may seem like a nearly impossible goal, but with a few thoughtful substitutions it can be easier than we imagined.

Sugar Free Diets

Our goal for eliminating sugar from our diets should be to get healthy first, if we lose a little weight along the way, that's great. Being a little overweight doesn't necessarily mean that we're not healthy. Weight loss diets don't work because our bodies want to hang on to every pound and will fight us every step of the way - that's how we evolved. We are the descendents of the people that survived the famines. It's in our DNA to conserve every last ounce of life giving energy. That's a pretty good strategy when we never know when this year's bumper crop will be followed by next year's drought.

However, when our bodies have to deal with a never-ending barrage of fat and sugar laden pseudo food, we don't stand a chance. Our only option is to kick the convenience food addiction and eat fresh, healthy, seasonal foods grown in nutrient-rich soil.

The Evil Empire's food industry has an iron grip on the general population and the government of the United States. South American and European governments still have a chance to legislate some changes but each year they seem to lose a little more ground.

The only way to win is with a grass roots movement that changes public eating habits one family at a time. Don't wait for the government to declare sugar a toxin, we need to eliminate it from our diets ourselves.

SUGAR-FREE DOES NOT MEAN CALORIE-FREE

It is important to remember that eliminating sugar from recipes does not necessarily eliminate calories. Remember, we won't be using any artificial sweeteners in these recipes, so whatever we do use as a sweetener will definitely have some calories and some of them even have some pretty hefty calorie counts.

DON'T PANIC!

We all need calories in order to function and to survive, however, what we need are the RIGHT calories from the RIGHT sources.

Sugar Free Recipes

This book is not intended to be a recipe book, but we want to show that eliminating sugar from our diets doesn't have to be difficult. There are thousands of recipes available. We are including just a "taste" from our sugar-free cookbook, "Break Your Sugar Addiction: Recipes With No Sugar, No Artificial Sweeteners, No Lies".

We have often found that many "sugar-free" recipes are loaded with artificial sweeteners. Although artificial sweeteners may be low calorie or calorie-free, we believe that anything artificial and/or highly processed is simply not good for us and is frequently harmful. Therefore, we feel it is best to define what we mean by sugar-free recipes. It is our intent to not only avoid standard table sugar but also avoid the use of any artificial sweeteners, or overly processed sweeteners of any kind, in our recipes and, most definitely, to avoid High Fructose Corn Syrup.

One thing that we have noticed is, when we start to cut down on highly sweetened foods, we become more sensitive to the naturally sweet tastes in most real foods.

That being said here's the list, from our cookbook, of the sweeteners we will, and won't, use:

SWEETENERS WE WON'T USE:

◊ Sugar, brown sugar, etc. - these recipes are, after all, sugar-free.

◊ Artificial sweeteners of any kind.

◊ Some "Natural" sweeteners that we believe are still too processed such as stevia and xylitol.

◊ Agave Nectar/Syrup - our research shows that agave nectar/syrup can be up to 90% fructose!

SWEETENERS WE WILL USE:

◊ **Corn syrup** - preferably non-GMO and definitely NOT High Fructose Corn Syrup. Why? Real corn syrup is 100% glucose.

Note: Our search for non-GMO corn syrup was a real challenge. So far, the only one we have found is Wholesome Sweeteners Organic Light Corn Syrup as certified by the [1]Non GMO Project.

You may have to use a name brand, like Karo (or Bee Hive in Canada), but when we checked with them, they confirmed that they do use GMO corn.

◊ **Honey** - be sure to get real, natural honey. There are a lot of impostors out there.

◊ **Dried fruits** - especially dates and prunes, but sparingly because drying fruits concentrates the sugar (fructose).

◊ **Unsweetened apple sauce** - preferably homemade, including the skin.

◊ **Grated carrots**

◊ **Grated beets** - the original sweetener and coloring for Red Velvet cakes.

◊ **Caramelized onions** - yes, they really are sweet! And, you can caramelize them without using oil.

◊ **Berries** - of all kinds, including, but not limited to, blueberries, strawberries, raspberries, etc.

◊ **Nuts** - whole, chopped or ground.

◊ **Maple syrup** - sparingly. Be sure to get real maple syrup, not maple flavoured syrup and definitely not pancake syrup.

The sweeteners we use do not have "empty" calories. Along with their calorie count, they also supply such things as fiber, vitamins, minerals, <u>nutrients and m</u>icronutrients.

1   http://www.nongmoproject.org/find-non-gmo/search-participating-products/search-by-name/?keyword=corn%20syrup

Breakfast

We've all heard it - breakfast is the most important meal of the day. And guess what? It's true! It's been found that if we skip breakfast, we're more likely to overeat later in the day and, possibly, in the evening, too.

Homemade, Sugar-Free, Granola

This is a staple in our household and we almost go into panic mode when we run out.

Yes, it is high calorie, but it also good for us. A serving of ½ cup, with a little non-dairy milk (almond milk, coconut milk, soy milk - all non-GMO, of course), is all that you need.

INGREDIENTS

4 cups rolled oats, old fashioned, not quick or minute
½ cup chia seeds
½ cup oat bran
½ cup ground flax seed
½ cup sunflower seeds
½ cup almonds, chopped
½ cup walnuts, chopped
½ teaspoon sea salt
½ cup honey
½ cup maple syrup
⅓ cup coconut oil
2 teaspoons ground cinnamon
1 ½ teaspoons vanilla extract (real vanilla, not the artificial stuff)
1 cup raisins
6 Medjool dates, pitted and chopped
1 tablespoon almonds, finely ground

DIRECTIONS

1. Pre-heat the oven to 325°F and lightly grease a large baking sheet.

2. Combine the oats, chia seeds, ground flax seeds, oat bran, sunflower seeds, almonds and walnuts in a large bowl.

3. In a small saucepan, mix together the salt, honey, maple syrup, coconut oil, cinnamon and vanilla. Over medium heat, bring the mixture to a boil and immediately remove from heat.

4. Allow the liquid mixture to cool for a couple of minutes and then pour it over the oat mixture and stir well to coat everything. Spread the mixture evenly on the greased baking sheet.

5. Bake at 325°F for 20 minutes. Remove from the oven and allow to cool.

6. While the granola is baking, chop up the Medjool dates and then toss them in the ground almonds to prevent them from sticking together.

7. Once the oatmeal mixture has cooled, break it up and add the raisins and dates. Toss together to mix well.

8. Store the completed granola in an airtight container. (We like to use a plastic Folgers Coffee container. It's the perfect size for this recipe and it's always good to recycle, too.)

Note: We wish we could tell you how long it keeps in an airtight container, but it never lasts very long in our house.

Servings: 16

Calories per ½ cup serving: 371

Simple Slow Cooker Oatmeal

Start this oatmeal recipe before bed and have it ready for breakfast the next morning. Dried cranberries can be substituted for fresh, but they often have added sugar. Raisins can also be substituted for the cranberries. The prunes add sweetness to the oatmeal so you may not want to add maple syrup as a garnish.

INGREDIENTS

1 cup old fashioned oats (NOT quick or minute oats)
1 cup cranberries, fresh or frozen
1 cup prunes, chopped
2 cups water
2 cups non-dairy milk
maple syrup, for garnish

DIRECTIONS

1. Lightly oil the crock of the slow cooker.

2. In the slow cooker, combine all the ingredients except the maple syrup. Stir gently and cover with the lid. Set the slower cook on low and cook for 7 to 8 hours.

3. Serve hot with a splash of maple syrup, if desired.

Servings: 4

Calories per serving: 259

Lunch

What's better than a nice bowl of soup for lunch? However, we have found that commercially produced canned soups contain a lot of stuff we don't want like MSG, a lot of salt and, yes, even sugar. Check the ingredients on canned soups carefully. Sometimes the sugar is hiding under a different name like glucose/fructose or High Fructose Corn Syrup.

Making our own soup doesn't have to be difficult and making it in a slow cooker takes it to another level of easy. Here's one of our favorites that's really tasty and low in calories to boot.

Salads are also a great choice for lunch but we may be, unintentionally, sabotaging our efforts with our choice of salad dressings. Many of the commercially produced salad dressings are amazingly high in calories and they often contain a lot of sugar and/or High Fructose Corn Syrup.

Any salad, of course, should contain lots of fresh leafy greens along with all of the other usual suspects, such as cucumber, radish, tomato, onion and more.

Making our own dressings is not difficult and it lets us control exactly what goes into it.

The best way to apply dressing to our salads is to add just a tablespoon or two to the salad in a mixing bowl and then toss to make sure everything gets covered. This way we'll use a lot less dressing, which equates to a lot fewer calories, than if we just poured it on.

Split Pea Soup

This tasty soup cooks all day which helps blend the flavors. It weighs in at only 199 calories per serving, so we can even enjoy a second helping if we want. As a bonus, this recipe is also vegan.

INGREDIENTS

2 cups split peas
4 medium carrots, chopped
2 cups cabbage, shredded
1 stalk celery, chopped
1 medium yellow onion, chopped
2 cloves garlic, minced
1 bay leaf
1 tablespoon salt
½ teaspoon pepper
6 cups vegetable broth, or water

DIRECTIONS

1. Lightly oil the crock of your slow cooker.

2. Layer ingredients in order listed, except for the vegetable broth, and don't stir it.

3. Gently pour the vegetable broth over the top, cover, set the slow cooker to low and cook for about 8 hours. The split peas should no longer be hard.

4. Remove the bay leaf and serve hot.

Servings: 8

Calories per serving: 199

Roasted Garlic Salad Dressing

Making our own salad dressings is not only easy, but it ensures that we get the freshest dressing without any added sugar or preservatives. And, it just plain tastes better!

Note: Instructions on how to roast the garlic follows.

Ingredients

2 heads roasted garlic, peeled
½ cup extra virgin olive oil
¼ cup apple cider vinegar, preferably with "The Mother"
2 tablespoons lemon juice, freshly squeezed
½ teaspoon kosher salt
1 teaspoon black pepper
1 tablespoon honey

Directions

1. Add all the ingredients to a food processor or blender and process until smooth.

2. Refrigerate until ready to serve and shake well before serving.

Servings: Approximately 12 - 2 Tablespoon servings

Calories per serving: 87

Hint: This dressing also makes a good marinade for grilled or roasted vegetables and even chicken or pork, if you eat meat.

How to Roast Garlic

1. Use complete heads of garlic.

2. With a sharp knife, carefully slice off the top of the garlic, just enough to expose the very top of each clove.

3. Drizzle each head with about 1 teaspoon of olive oil, trying to make sure that each of the cloves gets some of the oil.

4. For roasting just a couple of heads, place each head in a ceramic ramekin and cover with foil.

5. For roasting several heads at one time, use a muffin tin and cover each head with foil.

6. For roasting a small number of heads, pre-heat a toaster oven to 400°F and roast the garlic heads for 30 - 45 minutes until they are soft and slightly browned.

7. For roasting a large number of head, pre-heat a regular oven to 400°F and roast the garlic heads, in a muffin tin, for 30-45 minutes until they are soft and slightly browned.

8. Allow them to cool. Once cool the roasted cloves should come out easily either by squeezing each clove or by peeling them.

Hint: When we make garlic toast, we just spread mashed, roasted garlic on the toast - no butter. It tastes great!

Dinner

We often think that we're not getting a lot of sugar in our diets when we eat dinner. Well, yes - and - no. It depends on what we're having for dinner and whether it's prepared fresh or comes prepackaged or frozen.

Here's two recipes from our book for items that we don't normally think contain sugar but often do.

For the individual pizzas, we don't use store bought pizza sauce and for the stir fry we don't use a commercially produced stir fry sauce. Both of those commercial sauces are often loaded with added sugars. These hidden sugars can turn what seems like a healthy meal into one that's not healthy at all.

Individual Pizzas

Homemade pizza is usually a Friday night treat at our house. Frequently we make our own pizza dough, but this recipe uses flour tortillas and is super easy to make.

Instead of using commercially made pizza sauce, just use canned tomato paste and add the spices separately. Check the ingredients on cans of tomato paste - most list only one ingredient - tomatoes. Pass on the tomato pastes that already have herbs added. Often those ones will also have added salt.

Note: When choosing the tortillas, look for ones that only have 4 or 5 ingredients - like flour, water, salt, etc. - names we can recognize and pronounce.

INGREDIENTS

- 2 10" flour tortilla
- 2 tablespoons tomato paste
- 2 teaspoons Italian spice
- 1 small tomato, thinly sliced
- 4 black olives, thinly sliced
- ¼ medium yellow onion, thinly sliced
- ¼ medium sweet bell pepper, thinly sliced
- 2 large mushrooms, thinly sliced
- 2 ounces mozzarella cheese, shredded

DIRECTIONS

1. Pre-heat the oven to 375°F and lightly grease a baking sheet.
2. Place the two tortillas on the baking sheet and bake for 3 minutes each side, then remove from oven and allow to cool. They should be slightly brown and just a little crisp.
3. On each tortilla, spread 1 tablespoon of tomato paste. Then split all of the remaining ingredients between each pizza (tortilla), ending with the mushrooms and then the shredded cheese.
4. Return the pizzas to the oven and bake at 375°F for approximately 10 to 15 minutes or until the cheese is melted and bubbly.
5. Remove from oven and transfer the pizzas to a cutting board. Allow to cool for a couple of minutes and then slice each pizza into four wedges using a pizza cutting wheel or a sharp knife.

Servings: 2

Calories per serving: 358

Vegetable Stir Fry

With all these veggies, this recipe makes for a satisfying and filling meal. Whichever version of the stir fry sauce is chosen, it's still a very low calorie option. Pair it with some organic brown rice. And, for those who eat meat, add 1-2 cups of pre-cooked chicken, pork or beef to the recipe just before it is done and cook only long enough to heat the meat through.

INGREDIENTS

    1 teaspoon olive oil
    1 medium yellow onion, halved and sliced
    4 cloves garlic, minced
    ½ inch fresh ginger, piece, minced
    2 medium carrots, cut into matchsticks
    2 stalks celery, sliced
    ¼ medium cabbage, sliced
    1 cup broccoli, chopped
    ½ large green bell pepper, chopped
    ½ large red bell pepper, chopped
    1 cup sugar snap peas
    1 medium zucchini, halved and sliced
    6 mushrooms, sliced
    1 cup sugar-free stir fry sauce (recipe follows)

DIRECTIONS

1. Over medium-high heat, heat the oil in a large wok or deep frying pan. Add the garlic and ginger and cook for a minute or two.

2. Add the onion, carrots and celery and stir fry for 4 to 5 minutes, then add the cabbage and the broccoli and stir fry for another 3 to 4 minutes.

3. Add all of the stir fry sauce and mix well. Cover and cook for 5 minutes.

4. Add the zucchini, peppers, mushrooms and sugar snap peas, stir and cover. Continue to cook for another 4-5 minutes.

5. Remove from heat and serve over rice.

Servings: 4

Calories per serving excluding Stir Fry Sauce: 117

Calories per serving with Stir Fry Sauce made with dates: 190

Calories per servings with Stir Fry Sauce made without dates: 157

Sugar-Free Stir Fry Sauce

Some of us like our stir fry sauce a little sweeter than others. In this recipe the dates, as well as the red pepper flakes, are optional. The dates, however, almost double the calorie count for this sauce. In addition to that there is, naturally, fructose in the dates and because the sauce is being blended smooth, a lot of the effect of the fiber in the dates is diminished. But don't panic, all the fiber in the vegetables that go into this stir fry meal will help to offset any negative effect from the fructose.

INGREDIENTS

2 cups vegetable broth
¼ cup soy sauce
3 tablespoons cornstarch
1 inch fresh ginger, piece, minced
4 cloves garlic, minced
2 Medjool dates, chopped (optional)
¼ teaspoon red pepper flakes, optional

DIRECTIONS

1. Combine all ingredients in a food processor and blend until smooth.

2. Add to stir fry recipes as instructed.

Servings: 4 - ½ cup servings

Calories per serving: 73 with dates, 40 without dates

Breads

Check the ingredients on most commercially produced breads and we'll often see not only sugar but High Fructose Corn Syrup as well. In addition to that there will be a host of other ingredients including such things as "dough enhancer", which can often be plaster of Paris - no that's not a misprint. Yes, the yeast needs something to feed on and in most cases that's usually sugar, but it doesn't need to be. Honey and maple syrup work just as well.

We make all of our bread in a bread machine and then bake it in a conventional oven. A three-pound recipe can be split into two one-and-a-half pound loaves and then baked in the oven. As far as we're concerned, that's the best of both worlds - let the bread machine do all the mixing, kneading and rising - but still enjoy fresh baked loaves and the aroma that fills the kitchen.

Hint: an oven with just the interior light on is the perfect temperature for allowing bread dough to rise.

Rye Bread (Bread Machine Method)

This is one of our favorite rye bread recipes and we have made it both with and without the caraway seeds. It makes a great sandwich bread and toasts well, too.

Ingredients

    2 cups water, warm
    2 teaspoons salt
    3 tablespoons oil olive
    ¼ cup honey
    2 cups unbleached all-purpose flour
    2 cups whole wheat flour
    1 cup rye flour
    1 tablespoon yeast
    1½ tablespoons caraway seed, optional

Directions

1. Add all ingredients, with the exception of the caraway seeds, to the bread pan in the order suggested by the bread machine manufacturer.

2. Select the dough setting and press start.

3. Add the caraway seeds at the "add-in" beep.

4. Remove the dough from bread machine and knead for 2-3 minutes on a lightly floured surface.

5. Divide dough in half and place in two lightly greased loaf pans. Cover each loaf pan with plastic.

6. Allow the bread dough to rise, in a warm place, for about an hour.

7. After the loaves have risen, bake at 350°F for 30 to 35 minutes or until the loaves are well browned and sound hollow when tapped on the bottom.

8. Remove the loaves from the oven and remove the loaves from the loaf tins (they should come out easily). Then allow the loaves to cool completely on a wire rack. Bread slices best when it is cool.

Servings: 24 (12 slices per loaf)

Calories per serving: 115

Whole Wheat Sunflower Seed Bread (Bread Machine Method)

The sunflower seeds give this bread a lovely nutty taste and the wheat bran adds additional fiber. This loaf freezes well and is good for both sandwiches and toasting.

INGREDIENTS

2 cups warm water
2 tablespoons dry buttermilk powder
3 tablespoons olive oil
4 tablespoons honey
2 teaspoons sea salt
3 cups whole wheat flour
1½ cups unbleached all-purpose flour
1 cup wheat bran
2½ teaspoons active dry yeast
½ cup sunflower seeds

DIRECTIONS

1. Add all ingredients, with the exception of the sunflower seeds, to the bread pan in the order suggested by the bread machine manufacturer.

2. Select the dough setting and press start.

3. Add the sunflower seeds at the "add-in" beep.

4. Remove the dough from bread machine and knead for 2-3 minutes on a lightly floured surface.

5. Divide dough in half and place in two lightly greased loaf pans. Cover each loaf pan with plastic.

6. Allow the bread dough to rise, in a warm place, for about an hour.

7. After the loaves have risen, bake at 350°F for 30 to 35 minutes or until the loaves are well browned and sound hollow when tapped on the bottom.

8. Remove the loaves from the oven and remove the loaves from the loaf tins (they should come out easily). Then allow the loaves to cool completely on a wire rack. Bread slices best when it is cool.

Servings: 24 (12 slices per loaf)

Calories per serving: 130

Granola Bars & Fruit

Commercially produced granola bars may tout "healthy" ingredients, but be sure to read the labels carefully. Many of the store-bought versions contain sugar and even - gasp - High Fructose Corn Syrup, not to mention other things we may not want to put in our bodies.

Let's look for the sweetness we crave directly from nature but with a little twist - frozen grapes.

Chewy Sugar-Free Granola Bars

...sy to make, sugar-free, no-bake recipe makes lovely, chewy granola bars. You can alter the add-ins (sunflower seeds, raisins, etc.) as long as the total equals one cup, so be sure to experiment to get the type and taste you want.

Note: Don't go overboard on these, even though they are really tasty. Like we said before - sugar-free does NOT mean calorie free. And, at 237 calories per bar, these should be reserved for a special treat.

INGREDIENTS

½ cup natural peanut butter, smooth or chunky
⅓ cup honey
¼ cup coconut oil
1 cup old fashioned oats
¼ cup sunflower seeds
¼ cup raisins
¼ cup pepitas (pumpkin seeds)
¼ cup chia seeds

DIRECTIONS

1. Lightly grease an 8" x 8" glass baking dish and set aside.
2. In a medium saucepan, combine the peanut butter, honey and coconut oil. Heat over medium-low heat and stir until all ingredients are melted and well combined.
3. Remove the saucepan from the heat and add in the remaining ingredients. Stir well with a wooden spoon and make sure all ingredients are well mixed.
4. Pour the mixture into the greased baking dish, using a silicone spatula to get all of the mixture out of the saucepan and to press the mixture firmly into the baking dish.
5. Chill for at least two hours. Cut the mixture into 16 equal squares. Gently remove them from the baking dish and wrap individually with plastic wrap.
6. Store the individually wrapped bars in the fridge or freezer. They will be very chewy if stored in the fridge and have a little more snap to them if stored in the freezer. Yes, they can be eaten frozen.

Servings: 16
Calories per serving: 185

Frozen Grapes

Okay, it just doesn't get any easier, or more delicious, than this. How many recipes are there that have only ONE ingredient and incredibly simple directions?

And, yes, we'll be getting fructose from the snack. After all, it is fruit. However, we'll also be getting it in its natural form along with the fiber - just as nature intended.

INGREDIENTS

1 bunch green seedless grapes (or more, or less - your choice)

DIRECTIONS

1. Wash the grapes and pat them dry.

2. Remove the grapes from the stalk and, in a single layer, place them on a baking sheet lined with wax paper.

3. Place them in the freezer for several hours.

4. Repackage individually frozen grapes in resealable plastic bags and place them back in freezer for convenient snacking.

Serving: That will depend on the number of grapes we eat.

Calories per serving: 1 cup of seedless grapes is about 110 calories.

Desserts

It may be difficult to make sweet, tasty desserts without sugar - but it's not impossible! Here are two recipes from our book that eliminate the sugar and yet keep all the taste.

Sugar-Free, Gluten-Free, Egg-Free, Oil-Free Strawberry Muffins

This recipe started as a way to eliminate sugar from a muffin recipe that we really liked and then evolved to cover a lot of scenarios that friends and family had been asking about. So we developed the recipe to also eliminate gluten, eggs and oil. The muffins are still wonderful and are also vegan.

Ingredients

- 1 tablespoon ground flax seed
- 4 tablespoons water
- ⅔ cup sorghum flour
- ⅔ cup chickpea flour
- 1 cup gluten free quick oats
- 1 tablespoon baking powder
- ½ teaspoon sea salt
- ½ teaspoon cinnamon
- 1 cup rice milk
- 3 tablespoons unsweetened apple sauce
- 1 teaspoon vanilla
- 1 cup strawberries, fresh or frozen, diced

Directions

1. Pre-heat oven to 350°F and grease a muffin tin (makes 12).

2. In a small bowl, combine the ground flax seed and water. Stir well and set aside. (This makes an egg substitute.)

3. In a large mixing bowl, combine the sorghum flour, chickpea flour, oats, baking powder, salt and cinnamon. Mix well.

4. In a separate bowl or measuring cup, combine the liquid stevia, rice milk, applesauce, vanilla and flax seed mixture. Stir well.

5. Stir the liquid mixture into the dry mixture and mix just enough so that the dry ingredients are well moistened. Then fold in the diced strawberries.

6. Divide the batter evenly between the 12 muffin cups.

7. Bake at 350°F for 30-35 minutes or until a toothpick inserted in the center comes out clean and muffins are slightly browned.

8. Remove the muffins from the oven and cool on a wire rack for about 10 minutes. Remove the muffins from the muffin tin and allow them to continue cooling on the wire rack.

9. Any leftover muffins will freeze well.

Servings: 12

Calories per serving: 90

Mixed Fruit Cobbler

Traditionally made fruit cobbler is often loaded with sugar. In this recipe we've replaced the sugar in the fruit mixture with finely chopped Medjool dates. We've also replaced the sugar in the topping with unsweetened applesauce. And, this recipe has the added convenience of being made in a slow cooker!

Either fresh or frozen fruit works well in this recipe. When purchasing frozen fruit make sure it has no sugar added, or just buy extra fruit when it is in season and freeze it yourself. If you are unable to find fresh red currants, you can substitute blueberries.

INGREDIENTS

3 cups peaches, 3-4 medium peaches, pitted and sliced
2 cups golden plums, 14-16 small plums, pitted and sliced
1 cup red currants, fresh
6 Medjool dates, finely chopped
4½ teaspoons cornstarch
1½ teaspoons lemon juice, fresh
1 teaspoon vanilla

BATTER

1 cup whole wheat flour
1 teaspoons baking powder
½ teaspoon baking soda
2 tablespoons flax seed, ground
⅔ cup applesauce, unsweetened
1 tablespoon olive oil
1 teaspoon vanilla
2 tablespoons almond milk

DIRECTIONS

1. Lightly oil the crock of your slow cooker.

2. **Fruit Filling:** In a large bowl, combine the peaches, plums, currants (or blueberries), dates, cornstarch, lemon juice and vanilla extract. Toss to mix well. Spoon into the slow cooker.

3. **Batter**: In a large bowl, combine the first five ingredients (the dry ingredients) and mix well. Make a well in the center of the flour mixture and add the applesauce, oil, vanilla and almond milk. Stir

well to create a smooth batter. Gently pour the batter over the fruit mixture.

4. Place the lid on the slow cooker and turn to High setting. Cook for about 4 hours. The topping should be fully cooked and the fruit filling should be bubbly.

5. Turn off the slow cooker, remove the lid and allow the cobbler to cool for 15 minutes before serving.

Servings: 8

Calories per serving: 192

Section 7 Recap

We've covered a lot of information, mostly about sugar, but also about how huge corporations put their profits ahead of everything else, including our health and safety. In this section we'll try to give a concise recap along with a few other bits and pieces of information that are important for us to know.

Sugar and the Evil Empire

SECTION 1 - HISTORY

In this section we covered a brief history of sugar and discovered that the craving for this sweet stuff was, in no small part, the driving force for many countries' explorations and colonizations. And, that sugar was largely responsible for the justification of the brutal slave trade.

SECTION 2 - MEDICAL

Being over weight or even a little fat is OK if you're otherwise healthy. The trick is that you are not going to be healthy if you eat the standard North American diet. No way, no how, because what you are eating does not contain the nutrients your body needs. And, if you live on processed food you are eating food like products, not actual food. Real, in season food, contains nutrients your body needs, nutrients that are stripped out during processing.

Solutions to our obesity epidemic include:

◊ Never consume soft drinks or fruit juice. Don't drink your calories!

◊ Eliminate convenience and packaged foods.

◊ Eliminate or at least cut down on meat consumption.

◊ Eat a primarily plant-based diet.

◊ Pay the extra for organic, in-season food that contains nutrients.

◊ Best solution: grow our own food and eat what's in season, then freeze, pickle, can or dehydrate any excess produce.

SECTION 3 - SUGAR ADDICTION

We found it kind of scary that sugar is as, or more, addictive than cocaine, according to some studies.

There are ways to break the addiction and a quick-read article on [1]Yahoo gives some great tips.

---

1   https://ca.shine.yahoo.com/blogs/healthy-living/12-tips-kicking-

SECTION 4 - CORPORATE COMPLICITY

It is disturbing how little corporations care about the health and wellbeing of their consumers. The only thing that truly matters to them is their bottom line.

Throughout history we have many examples of such disregard for safety and health matters with many other products, not just sugar.

Here's a few examples of some of the things that corporations have told us are safe, even when they knew they weren't:

◊ Lead - in paint, in gasoline, used as solder in food cans, used as solder in water pipes. Some, but not all, of these issues have been addressed but only as the result of public pressure.

◊ [2]Cigarettes

◊ Agent Orange - a great disservice to those who were already put in harms way.

◊ Monsanto's Roundup

◊ These are just a few examples ...

SECTION 5 - LIVING WITH SUGAR

In Section 5 we explore just how ubiquitous sugar is in our daily lives, even right down to our vocabulary. We offer suggestions and resources for dealing with both the obvious and hidden sources of sugar that we live with every day.

SECTION 6 - COOKING WITHOUT SUGAR

Cooking without sugar is not only possible but tasty, too. In Section 6 we supply a few recipes to help get us thinking about sugar-less cooking possibilities.

---

refined-sugar-habit-173400965.html
2   http://en.wikipedia.org/wiki/Brown_%26_Williamson

We Need To Get Angry, Very Angry

Here's how we can make a difference:

◊ Refuse to allow a few corporations to control our food supply. We can accomplish this by voting with our dollars (We've said this several times throughout this book because we truly believe it can, and does, work.)

◊ March against Monsanto - the poster child for GMOs (Find your local [3]March Against Monsanto group and join!)

◊ Help spread the word. It seems like we're making headway but there are still so many people out there that haven't heard about the dangers of sugar (in all it's forms).

◊ Visit the Terra Novian Website at http://www.terranovian.com We created this website in order to bring together all the critical information each and every one of us needs to know, not just about sugar but about GMOs, the financial crisis, climate change and more.

Things We Need To Know

◊ Our [4]children will not live as long as we will and that has a lot to do with sugar and chronic diseases. This is the first generation where children do not have the same, or better, life expectancy as their parents.

◊ We are becoming [5]infertile.

◊ Processed food are not safe, not just because of the additives but because of the [6]missing nutrients.

◊ Corporations are fighting [7]GMO labelling with big budgets and we need to ask why.

3   http://www.march-against-monsanto.com/p/blog-page_5.html
4   http://www.aspeninstitute.org/policy-work/health-biomedical-science-society/health-stewardship-project/principles/we-shouldn
5   http://www.dailymail.co.uk/femail/article-1275879/The-infertility-timebomb-Are-men-facing-rapid-extinction.html
6   http://www.washingtonpost.com/lifestyle/food/processed-foods-the-problem-probably-isnt-whats-in-them-its-whats-not-in-them/2014/04/24/93e60a4e-c3f2-11e3-b574-f8748871856a_story.html
7   http://www.huffingtonpost.com/2013/10/29/food-giants-pour-millions_n_4175592.html

Raise Your Voice

We hope you are convinced that sugar is much worse than we thought and that the processed food branch of the Evil Empire has known it all along.

We can't stress it enough. If you believe, as we do, that corporations don't care about anything except making a profit, it's time for us to all raise our voices and let them know we won't take it any more.

It's also time to hurt them where they will feel it the most, in their bottom lines. Stop buying their garbage, it is making us fat and sick. STOP IT.

If you own shares in any fast food or proceed food companies, sell them. If you own mutual funds that own shares in food companies, sell them. If you are a parent, get involved with the school board and demand the schools serve real food and dump the junk.

Unfortunately, food is just one small part of what is going terribly wrong with our world. Most people are just vaguely aware that some things are not quite right but they are not willing to dig any deeper. When you try to tell them they stick their fingers in their ears and say, "la la la la". It's too bad but you just can't fix stupid.

There are many issues that demand your attention and your involvement but unless you know they exist you can't do anything about them. You owe it to yourself and your family to find out. Click the link below to take the first step.

http://www.terranovian.com

Suggested Viewing & Reading

If you have not already done so you need to watch the two YouTube videos from Dr. Lustig - [8]*Sugar, The Bitter Truth* and [9]*Fat Chance: Fructose 2.0*.

He presents the science behind what you have read here. We have also provided the links to them and a whole lot more on the Terra Novian web site.

If you're ready for some more in depth reading check out the books *Fat Chance: Beating the Odds Against Sugar, Processed Food, Obesity, and Disease* by Dr. Robert Lustig and *Salt Sugar Fat: How the Food Giants Hooked Us* by Michael Moss.

And, of course, there's Google. Once you know what to look for you will find thousands of references to the subjects we've covered in this book.

---

8   http://www.youtube.com/watch?v=dBnniua6-oM
9   http://www.youtube.com/watch?v=ceFyF9px20Y

Section 8 Before You Go

Thank you for purchasing our book. The new popularity of Indy publishing is a wonderful opportunity for everyone to express their ideas but unfortunately there are always the quick buck artists that threaten to spoil a good thing.

With every book we publish we try to get a little better and give our loyal readers true value for money. If you enjoyed this book please take a moment to post a review on the web site you used for purchase and any other blogs or book review sites you belong to.

Meet The Authors

Since committing to a vegetarian lifestyle almost two years - and several pounds - ago, Geoff and Vicky Wells have continued to research how food affects our health.

This research naturally led to investigating the storm that is brewing over our increasing sugar consumption, High Fructose Corn Syrup (HFCS) and Genetically Modified Organisms (GMOs).

This led, of course, to research on agribusiness and food corporations and the realization that the Evil Empire actually did exist and that much of their greed and manipulations can be traced back in history to the rise in the production, supply and consumption of sugar.

Both Geoff and Vicky are eager to share what they've learned not only in this book but also on their Terra Novian website. A website that is dedicated to bringing together all the things we need to know about how our world, our very lives, are being altered by the machinations of the Evil Empire.

If you want to be sure we are real people you can visit http://geoffandvickywells.com. It's mostly a lot pages that say "coming soon" but one day we will find the time to add some more content.

Please Review

Independent (Indy) authors rely to a great extent on word of mouth and peer reviews to promote the books we write. We are very aware that the quality of writing and editing varies a great deal from author to author.

We don't always get it right but we do try very hard to give you a quality product at a fair price. And we write every word ourselves - we never outsource our books to third world authors.

We would very much appreciate it if you would leave a review of this book on the site from which you purchased it and also on web sites like Good Reads (https://www.goodreads.com) and Shelfari (http://www.shelfari. com)

If you believe, as we do, that everyone needs to know how the corporate food empires are poisoning us and our children we urge you to use the power of social media to blog, twitter, facebook etc to spread the word.

If you enjoyed this book you may also enjoy the companion cookbook. Lots more recipes without any sugar, artificial sweeteners or lies.

Break Your **Sugar Addiction**

POISON

Recipes With NO Sugar Artificial Sweeteners Lies

A Terra Novian Recipe Book by Geoff & Vicky Wells

Other Books You May Enjoy

After spending most of our lives eating meat we made the decision to become vegetarians, not because we don't like meat but because the chemicals added by Big Food make it no longer healthy to do so.

We also discovered that animal cruelty laws do not apply to food animals. We could not, in good conscience, be a party to the pain and suffering animals must endure in our modern food factories.

Our decision resulted in a learning process for us as we discovered the challenges, difficulties, tastes and delights of becoming vegetarians. We have documented our discoveries in a series of books under the collective banner of "The Reluctant Vegetarians". We hope you enjoy the books and join us for some of the best food you have ever tasted.

A Guide to Juicing, Raw Foods & Superfoods

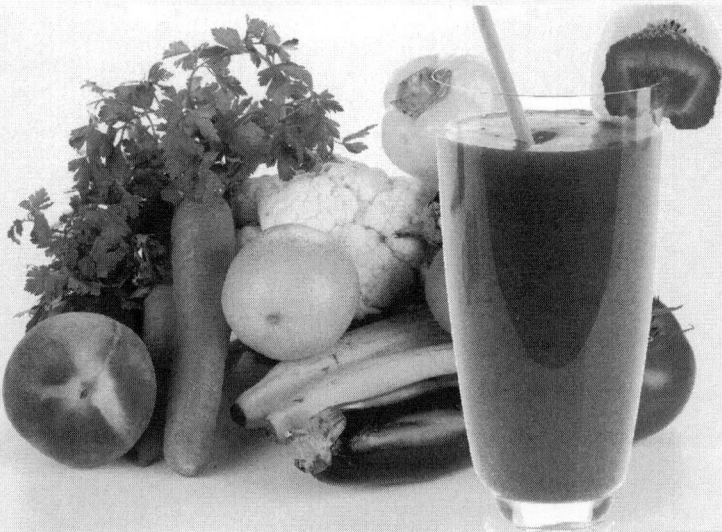

A Guide to Juicing, Raw Foods & Superfoods

Eat a Healthy Diet & Lose Weight

Geoff & Vicky Wells

The Reluctant Vegetarians

http://bit.ly/SeoZAs

SUPER 3 DAY DETOX SOUP & SMOOTHIE PLAN

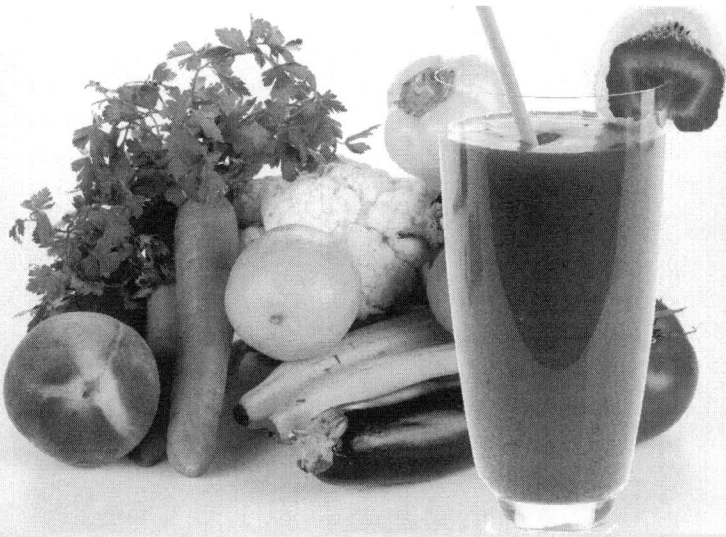

Super 3 Day Detox Soup & Smoothie Plan

How To Cleanse Your Body With Vegetable Smoothies, Slow Cooker Soups & Fresh Fruits

Geoff & Vicky Wells

The **Reluctant Vegetarians**

http://bit.ly/1pTkObM

**OUR FAVORITE DETOX & WEIGHT LOSS
SLOW COOKER RECIPES**

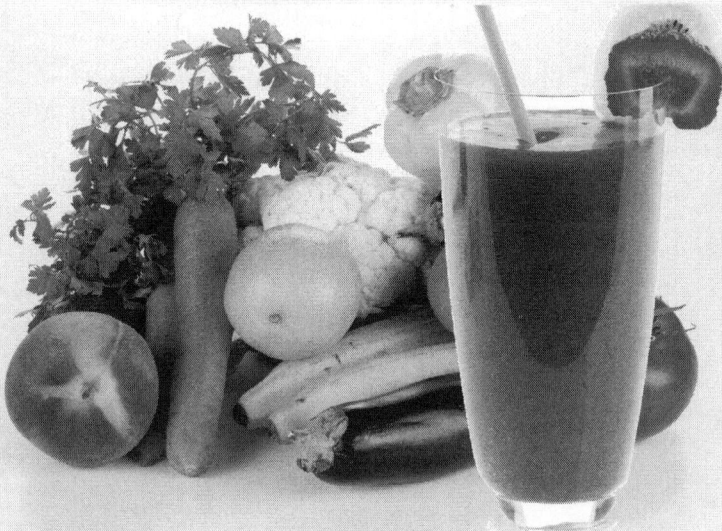

Our Favorite Detox & Weight Loss Slow Cooker Recipes

Look Great~Get Healthy~Lose Weight

Geoff & Vicky Wells

The **Reluctant Vegetarians**

http://bit.ly/1pTkY2Q

SECTION 8 INDEX

Index

A

Acetyl-CoA 36
Addiction 41, 62, 63, 66, 67, 68, 69, 122, 124, 150
Adenine 39
Adenosine triphosphate 36
Africa 15, 16, 17, 33
Agave 88, 124
Agricultural Adjustment Act 23
Alcohol 37, 38, 103, 104, 110
Amygdala 40
Ancestors 47, 49, 50, 54, 97, 100, 109, 112
Arabia 33

B

Baking 98
Barley 88
Bee 116
Belly fat 39, 54, 64, 66, 102
Big Food 81, 82, 84, 85, 97, 159
Bliss 72
Blood Sugar 5, 30
Breakfast 60, 100, 112, 113, 114, 126, 129
Brown Rice Syrup 89
Brown Sugar 89
Butz, Earl 23

C

Calorie 5, 6, 28, 33, 34, 35, 36, 37, 38, 40, 50, 58, 59, 62, 64, 78, 84, 86, 90, 96, 99, 103, 110, 123, 124, 125, 127, 128, 129, 130, 131, 132, 135, 136, 137, 139, 140, 142, 143, 146, 148, 150
Canada 19, 20, 33, 87, 90, 117, 125
Cancer 29, 46, 47, 49, 54, 55, 109
Cane Juice 89, 91
Cane Sugar 89
Carbohydrates 5, 30, 34, 38, 87
Carbon dioxide 34
Cargill 73
Carob Syrup 89
Chronic Kidney Disease 21
Coca Cola 71, 73
Confectioner's Sugar 89
Convenience Food 106
Corn Sweetener 90

Printed in Great Britain
by Amazon.co.uk, Ltd.,
Marston Gate.